More praise for *The Health of Nations*

'This is a biting and insightful book on what is wrong with the political economy of the world today that so much goes wrong with our health systems. Sharply written and informative in the best Zed tradition!'
Gita Sen, Centre for Public Policy, Indian Institute of Management

'Inequality, whether of wealth or power, undermines our best efforts to provide effective support to communities in their quest for better health. Mooney challenges neoliberal assumptions and through elegant case studies demonstrates how we can improve what we do through real community involvement in making decisions about health according to the values that matter.'
Stephen Leeder, director, The Menzies Centre for Health Policy, ANU and University of Sydney

'Many social scientists and activists have long felt extremely frustrated by a paradigm which links health care closely to the market – a market that is supposed to be free of corporate power. While exposing the misdeeds of big corporations and their clientelistic governments, Mooney's book indicates how much can be achieved by, first, promoting communitarianism in a principled and rational way and, second, listening to the concerns of the people being served by health care, not just hospital managers or those in the medical profession.'
Amiya Bagchi, Institute of Development Studies Kolkata

About the author

Gavin Mooney is based in Tasmania, Australia. He has worked as a health economist for 40 years and held academic positions in Scotland, Scandinavia, South Africa and Australia. In 2009 he was given an honorary doctorate by the University of Cape Town as 'one of the founding fathers of health economics'. He has published widely with over 20 books to his name. Gavin has also acted as a consultant to the WHO and the OECD. Equity is a key research focus. In recent years he has become particularly interested in the impact of poverty and inequality on health and of neoliberalism on society's power structures and health-care systems. These concerns inform his *Challenging Health Economics*, published in 2009. He is also an advocate for using community values through citizens' juries in health care (see www.gavinmooney.com).

The Health of Nations

Towards a New Political Economy

Gavin Mooney

With a preface by Vicente Navarro

Zed Books

LONDON & NEW YORK

The Health of Nations: Towards a New Political Economy was first published in 2012 by
Zed Books Ltd, 7 Cynthia Street, London N1 9JF, UK
and Room 400, 175 Fifth Avenue, New York, NY 10010, USA

www.zedbooks.co.uk

Copyright © Gavin Mooney 2012
Preface © Vicente Navarro 2012

The right of Gavin Mooney to be identified as the author of this work has been asserted
by him in accordance with the Copyright, Designs and Patents Act, 1988

Designed and set in Warnock Pro with Din display by Kate Kirkwood
Index by John Barker
Cover designed by Rogue Four Design
Printed and bound in Great Britain by CPI Group (UK) Ltd, Croydon CR0 4YY

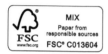

Distributed in the USA exclusively by Palgrave Macmillan, a division of
St Martin's Press, LLC, 175 Fifth Avenue, New York, NY 10010, USA

A catalogue record for this book is available from the British Library
Library of Congress Cataloging in Publication Data available

ISBN 978 1 78032 060 1 hb
ISBN 978 1 78032 059 5 pb

Contents

Acknowledgements

The writing of this book has been a most interesting experience for me. Certainly before setting out I was aware of many of the issues that I cover. How could it be otherwise? Yet some of the things I discovered as I researched the book have shocked me. Adopting a political economy stance throughout has made me realise much more clearly and strongly than when I started just how badly the world is coping with ill-health. This is a world rich in resources. It is also staggeringly unequal and inequitable.

The extent of research and debate around economic structural issues regarding how this planet is run is remarkably limited. Yet that matters, especially when for the great mass of humanity it is clearly being run very badly. The most obvious example of this planetary mismanagement is global warming, but the way we organise the production and distribution of pharmaceuticals, the machinations of our undemocratic 'global' institutions and the corporatisation of governments are also examples of the corruption of power and the dereliction of any global sense of decency. I have also felt some sadness that my own discipline of health economics has not done more to try to build that better world, and if I have upset my health economist colleagues with some of my criticisms then let me apologise here. I only seek to spur us all to better things!

I have also been hard on the medical profession in places. Yet I have enormous respect for medicine – it is a truly noble calling – and for those caring doctors who day after day move mountains to try to help their patients. My concern is with the politicking that corporate medicine and particularly medical associations indulge in.

There are all sorts of ideas and thoughts built into this book that have been gleaned from various places and people. I have learned so much from Jon Ataguba, Amiya Bagchi, David Coburn, Dennis Eggington, Bob Evans, Karen Gerard, Lucy Gilson, Geoff Harcourt, Steve Jan, Uffe Juul Jensen, Ivar Sonbo Kristiansen, Steve Leeder, Miles Little, Maureen Mackintosh, Alan Maynard, Di McIntyre, Michael Moodie, Narayana, Vicente Navarro, Jan Abel Olsen, Tom Rice, Glenn Salkeld, Jes Sogaard, Ted Wilkes, Virginia Wiseman and Alex Wodak. Thank you all.

I also want to thank at another level. Like most people I suppose I look for inspiration from others. In writing this book I harbour some thoughts that it might just help in some small way to bring about a better world. In believing that it might, I have been inspired by others, friends and colleagues, who not only try to bring about a better world but succeed. So my thanks to Amiya Bagchi, Nkwame Cedile, Dennis Eggington, Bob Evans, Uffe Juul Jensen, Di McIntyre, Michael Moodie, Grant Mooney, Rachel Mooney, Narayana, Vicente Navarro, Tinashe Njanji and Alex Wodak.

Ken Barlow at Zed Books has been great. It was Ken who believed enough in my early ideas to see how these might be shaped into a readable, useful book. He pushed me to think in terms of case studies. That worked for me as an author. I hope it does for the reader. He also did an excellent job of editing and improved some rather ugly sentences. Thanks Ken. The copyediting by Mike Kirkwood was not only thorough but inspiring and so much in the spirit of the book.

My biggest debt, however, is to my wife, Del Weston, who was the real inspiration for me in writing this book. Constantly supportive and encouraging, Del has been working on her PhD on the political economy of global warming for much of the time I have been writing. I learned so much from her about global warming and political economy. I'd like to think too I have learned much about how to be supportive and to fight for what I believe in. You are a 'bonnie fechter', Del. Thanks my honey.

Preface
Vicente Navarro

We are witnessing in these times the consequences of public policies that have been put forward by the major international centres and governments of what are usually referred to as 'developed countries'. These policies were initiated by President Ronald Reagan in the United States and Prime Minister Margaret Thatcher in Great Britain, subsequently followed by many other governments and then reproduced by the International Monetary Fund and the World Bank, and, in Europe, by the European Central Bank, the European Commission and the European Council. The major characteristics of those policies were the deregulation of finance, commerce and the labour market, with a corresponding decline in wages and social protection and the privatisation of public services. As President Reagan indicated, 'government is not the solution, but rather is the problem'. It is worth stressing that this anti-state position was clearly selective, particularly targeted against the public and social programmes that had been implemented since World War II and which had improved the lives and well-being of millions of people all over the world. Otherwise, the state was transformed to become an enormous welfare provider for parasitic institutions like the military industries, which require wars in order to sustain themselves, and speculative finance, as we have seen recently in the large bailouts of financial centres by the governments on both sides of the North Atlantic. The US and European Union transferred enormous sums of money to the very financial institutions responsible for the current recession, which may become another Great Depression.

These policies – usually referred to as neoliberalism – have had an enormous negative impact on the well-being, quality of life and health of the populations of developed and developing countries. Inequality has grown to an unprecedented level. We must go back to the beginning of the twentieth century, before the Great Depression, to see similar levels of income and wealth inequalities. It is worth expressing that those inequalities existed not only among countries, but within each country. The impact of these neoliberal policies on the well-being, quality of life and health of the popular classes has been enormously harmful. And what is even more overwhelming is that in spite of these consequences, they are stubbornly put forward by those governments that have made this austerity a principle and centerpiece of their interventions.

The awareness of this reality explains the surge of interest in an area of knowledge usually referred to as the social determinants of health. This is indeed a positive step but an insufficient one. Scholarship needs to take one step further and look at the political context of neoliberalism with consequences and possible solutions, which are especially urgent in the parts of the world where the majority of people live. In fact, it is in these parts of the world, which have long suffered under these policies for long periods of time, that new developments are occurring that represent a break with neoliberalism and that point the way of change. It is urgent that those new experiences be studied and that we see their relevance to other settings.

This book, *The Health of Nations*, is a positive addition to this new line of inquiry. Written in clear and concise language and free of academic jargon, it explains with utmost rigor what is going on, why it is going on and how it affects the health and quality of life in today's world. It also offers important and viable solutions.

The reader will be absorbed from the first to the last page. This important book contains a wealth of information that he or she needs to be able to dismantle the huge ideological construct trying to cover up the enormous amounts of oppression and exploitation in today's world.

It could not have been written by a better author than Professor Gavin Mooney. Dr Mooney is internationally known for his most strict and scholarly rigor and discipline combined with an unyielding commitment to improving the health and well-being of populations. This book is not only immediately relevant, it will become a classic. It undoubtedly will be a point of reference in the existing literature aimed at a fuller understanding of our world in order to change it.

Vicente Navarro
Professor of Health Policy
Johns Hopkins University

To Del

PART I / Introduction

Introduction:
neoliberalism kills

There is something desperately wrong with our health-care systems and with our societies when, in this amazingly rich world, there is still so much ill health and premature death. What is at least as wrong is that there are such enormous differences between the rich and the poor. Hunger is of endemic proportions; obesity too. But the latter gets so much more attention as it is a disease of the affluent who can corner the market for sympathy and health-care resources. There are too few headlines in hunger.

This state of affairs can be summed up in all sorts of ways. One particularly telling way is provided by the philosopher Thomas Pogge (2008):

> Many more people – some 360 million – have died from hunger and remediable diseases in peacetime in the 20 years since the end of the Cold War than have perished from wars, civil wars, and government repression over the entire 20th century. And poverty continues unabated, as the official statistics amply confirm: 963 million human beings are chronically undernourished, 884 million lack access to safe water, and 2,500 million lack access to basic sanitation. 2,000 million lack access to essential medicines. 924 million lack adequate shelter and 1,600 million lack electricity. 774 million adults are illiterate. 218 million children are child laborers. Roughly one third of all human deaths, 18 million annually, are due to poverty-related causes, straightforwardly preventable through better nutrition, safe drinking water, cheap re-hydration packs, vaccines, antibiotics, and other medicines. People of color, females, and the very young are heavily overrepresented among the global poor, and hence also among those suffering the staggering effects of severe poverty. Children under five account for over half or 9.2 million of the annual death toll from poverty-related causes. The overrepresentation of females is clearly documented.

Specifically with respect to health care, there is the grotesque situation where the poorer a country, the more likely it is to have a smaller proportion of its health-care resources in the public sector. Yet having to pay for health care, which is much more likely in the private sector, increasingly dominates poor countries' health-care systems, while this privatisation of health care in poor countries continues to be encouraged by the rich West and global institutions like the World Bank. In India, for example, little more than 20 per cent of the spend on health care is in the public sector.

The fact that poverty kills is clear, well known and easily understood. Yet so little is done about it. The fact that inequality kills is also clear, less well known and not so easily understood. Even less is done about that. And inequality is morally disgraceful. It could be addressed; it should be addressed. Yet, for example, South Africa, freed from the chains of apartheid in 1994, is more unequal today than it was then and is now one of the most unequal countries in the world.

Inequality within countries is also growing, with truly obscene levels of incomes in many Western countries – certainly in comparison to the incomes of the poor in low and middle-income countries, but also to the poor in their own countries.

Astonishingly, in Australia a very minor use of the tax system in the 2011 budget to redistribute income from the rich to the poor (after years of movement in the opposite direction and a growing gap between rich and poor) was met with cries of 'class warfare' and 'the politics of envy'.

We are soothed by the appearance of efforts to do better. At a global level there are the Millennium Development Goals, the WHO commissions on Macroeconomics and Health and on Social Determinants of Health, and the World Trade Organization's Doha Agreement to reduce world poverty. But success? There is some movement but it is tiny, as the rich world gets more obese and more unhealthy because of its own greed. The Doha Agreement, originally launched in 2001 with great fanfare and the intent to reduce world poverty, is still being negotiated ten years on. Even if it ever were to be enacted, according to best estimates it would produce greater benefits for rich countries than for poor (Hertel and Winters 2006).

These international global institutions are not genuinely world bodies in that they do not represent world citizenry. They are controlled by governments, and only the governments of a few rich nations. In turn these governments are often swayed by large corporations who seek to maximise their profits on the basis of a market system that is built on the false premise that this maximises the public good.

Yet worship at the altar of the market, and especially the neoliberal market in the wake of the fall of the Berlin Wall, is seldom seriously challenged. The Communism of the former Eastern Bloc is gone. Its departure is welcome, but the hegemony of neoliberalism that has replaced it is most unwelcome on a number of fronts. Here I focus on its perpetuating and fostering of ill health.

This book concentrates its criticism of macroeconomic and global economic systems on the political economy of neoliberalism. This is the form of capitalism that was ushered in in the late 1970s by President Reagan in the US and Prime Minister Thatcher in the UK, and heralded by the Washington Consensus. It is explored at greater length in Chapter 3. While the focus on that form of capitalism is appropriate in examining most of the issues in this book, since they primarily relate to modern times, capitalism has existed ever since the dawn of the industrial revolution in the eighteenth century, and some of today's current ills – particularly global warming but also the continuing impact of colonialism – have their origins in those earlier times.

We know that solidarity and social cohesion are good for health and that individualism and inequality are not. Yet it is the latter that neoliberalism fosters. There remains debate as to whether neoliberalism fosters economic growth, since comparison with the counter-factual is difficult – and even more difficult when it comes to the impact on health. Whether economic growth is good for health also remains debatable. Poverty is bad, so lifting people out of poverty is good for their health. But the distribution of the benefits of economic growth are all too often skewed to the rich; 'trickle down' has been exposed as a myth. There is also evidence that how a society uses and organises its resources may have a greater impact on health than simply the level of those resources. The rich get the diseases of affluence, the poor of deprivation.

Inequality seems to breed ill-health in society as a whole. It is those at the bottom, however, who really suffer – in terms of both health and humiliation. What is perhaps most humiliating for them is the seeming indifference of the rich to the situation of the poor.

Debates about health all too often centre on health care rather than the so-called social determinants of health – poverty, inequality, housing, transport, education, et cetera. This is especially true at a governmental level, where ministries of health are ministries of only health care. And too often, in the West at least, they are not about health care so much as illness care, their services dominated by hospitals. The idea of the social determinants of health, while given a boost by Sir Michael Marmot's WHO Commission, has been slow to percolate through to health policy.

Neoliberalism brings with it low taxes. It also breeds freer movement of money and resources across national boundaries. The extent to which governments in a neoliberal world are any longer prepared to use taxes to redistribute income from rich to poor is severely limited. If the UK gets out of line on, say, its company taxes and becomes less attractive than other countries to profit-hunting industrial investors, then – so the argument goes – the UK will lose out on investment and thus on jobs. Similarly, seeking to increase levels of income tax, and especially to make income tax more progressive, is seen as likely to scare the brightest and best into moving overseas. There is a race to the bottom on tax rates, with company taxes declining markedly over the last couple of decades. Thus we learn that 'The OECD average top (federal) statutory company tax rate fell from 44 per cent in 1985 to 31 per cent in 2004, on a GDP-weighted basis' (Kelly and Graziani 2004: 24).

It was not always thus. I recall Conservative governments in the UK, in my early years, having a real concern to take care of the poor and disadvantaged – and that was when we were all much poorer than we are now. Between the West and the others on the planet today there is a massive barrier; and this despite the fact that our TVs allow us to see and almost smell the devastation wreaked by poverty across the globe – in Haiti, in so many African countries, or in the wake of the 2004 Boxing Day tsunami. The words of the Turkish writer Orhan Pamuk (2001) ring true: 'The Western world is scarcely aware of this overwhelming feeling of humiliation that is experienced by most of the world's population.'

The freedom of movement of labour internationally from poor to rich countries is problematic, as those who move are those with skills. Rich countries continue to steal doctors and nurses from, for example, sub-Saharan Africa. Again, bearing out the indifference highlighted by Pamuk, it is remarkable how little concern is expressed by governments and medical associations in the West at this process of adding to the global divide – especially in health.

The growth imperative – or the growth fetishism as Hamilton (2003) has called it – that drives this is born of neoliberalism. That economic thinking may well result in faster economic growth (although that remains unproven), but to be conducive to improved population health it needs to be accompanied by reductions in poverty and in inequalities. The neoliberal panacea of the 'trickle down' effect, the 'rising tide that lifts all boats', has not stood up to examination.

The behaviour of the pharmaceutical industry – 'Big Pharma' – and the way it exercises power over doctors and governments are deeply concerning. These issues have been exposed, but again what needs to be recognised is that these companies are acting according to the rules of the market place. Their goal is profit maximisation, not health maximisation.

This book is not intended in any sense as an attack on doctors as doctors, nor on medicine as a discipline. But when medical associations and the medical profession become political I have concerns. In individual countries the medical associations dominate debates about much more than medicine, and seek to speak with authority on matters of health. All too often governments treat them as spokespersons for the health of the population. In reality they are the doctors' trade unions.

While the problem here may be created by the medical profession, and more particularly by their associations when they take on a political role, it can only be solved by governments being more ready to see these associations for what they are – organisations whose first and foremost interest is the well-being of the medical profession. Governments need to be prepared, instead, to serve the public whose health is at stake.

Decision making regarding resources for health must be understood as the exercise of power at two levels: health care and society. The power in health care currently rests all too much with the medical profession and the pharmaceutical industry, and all too little with the citizenry. That this needs to change is a major theme of this book.

The extent to which the medical profession is in the pockets of the big pharmaceutical companies is extraordinary, with massive amounts of money being used by the industry to 'persuade' doctors to prescribe their products. This is done openly, in the sense that we all know it happens – and yet somehow the practice and the culture have become acceptable. We know too that pharmaceutical companies have ghost-written articles for journals and then paid doctors to put their names to them, and this practice continues despite having been exposed. We know that drug trials that are funded by the industry are more likely to come up with results that are favourable to the product, but such funding remains the main source for researchers wanting to test the effectiveness of drugs. Too many academics have sold out to 'Big Pharma'.

So many societies today – and the trend continues – are dominated by the market and large corporations. Very little power within so-called democracies rests with the people. Australia, for example, has seen the power of the mining industry exerted on government policy recently, when the industry's $20 million campaign to stop a mining tax on excess profits denied the government $10 billion in annual revenue which had been earmarked to provide, inter alia, better health services. Another example is the influence of industry in seeking to undermine policy on global warming in many countries.

The problems that arise in dealing with these two issues – the dominance of the medical profession and the pharmaceutical industry in health care, and the dominance of corporate power in society – are the centrepiece of this book. It examines the reasons why we need to change, as well as what we need to change *to*.

The book also deals with the fact that my own sub-discipline of health economics – which in many ways ought to be well placed to analyse what is, in our terms, the inefficient and inequitable use of scarce resources – fails to do so. We have been caught like rabbits in the headlights of neoliberalism and cannot see an alternative. We have followed the doctors down the micro-clinical road and viewed health-care systems as only consequentialist – and very narrowly consequentialist, where nothing counts but health. We have not stopped to ask citizens what they want from health-care systems, perhaps because we are so tied to neoclassical economics that we do not see citizens *qua* citizens – only consumers. Our neglect of the social determinants of health is astonishing.

Can the changes be made? They need to be made and some suggestions are put forward. If I can convince the reader that the current organisation and financing of health care (like the economic basis of many of our societies) is bad for the health of the population, then the question of how to bring about change will become the key focus of health-policy debates. Currently it is not. That shift of focus is my main target in writing this book.

Map of the book

The book is in six parts. Between the introduction (Part I) and the conclusion (Part VI) there are case studies of the bad and the good, and some thoughts on solutions to the global problems of ill-health and premature death. These are massive problems and that is where we have started. The book does not dwell on them. Most readers will know of them already – though it is worth stopping and recognising anew just how big they really are, and how unfair, given the wonderfully good health of some and the miserable health of others.

Part II looks at why things are so bad. It examines policies on health care and on health and why these are failing. While it would be wrong to argue that there is a single cause of the malaise, I place much of the explanation for not doing better at the door of neoliberalism. This form of capitalism – which has increasingly dominated the world stage over the last 30 years and sees the market as the solution to virtually all the world's problems – has direct economic consequences for health, but also broader social ones. It breeds inequality and individualism and discourages a sense of community and feelings of compassion. I have also examined the way it dominates our global institutions.

In Part III there is a series of case studies which serve to exemplify many of the points made in Part II. Some of these are country-specific; others relate to issues or organisations. The US fear of socialism in Obama's reforms is illustrated. The attempts – by the current coalition government, but also by Labour governments before it – to bring the market into the UK's National Health Service (NHS) are detailed. In the South African case study the miserable state of health and of health care in that country are highlighted, together with the continuing post-apartheid inequality in health, health care and society as a whole consequent on the ANC's embrace of neoliberalism. The 'victim-blaming' policies in health promotion in Australia are presented against a background of the corporatisation of health policy. That corporatisation theme is carried over into Chapter 9, which sets out the David and Goliath battle between the small town of Yarloop in Western Australia and the corporate giant Alcoa. The case study also shows how a corporation gets backing from government in the interests of economic growth and also worms its way into influence within the groves of academe.

The last two case studies in Part III are on the pharmaceutical industry and global warming. While many readers will already be aware that the pharmaceutical industry is very powerful with respect to both doctors and governments, what I hope to do is to exemplify just how far that industry is prepared to go in pursuit of profits. On global warming I show how capitalism and more recently neoliberalism are responsible in large part for global warming, and also that they do not offer a solution.

Part IV looks for solutions to the problems of global ill health. It argues that we need a new political economy of health. It presents a communitarian model which provides a way forward to a more egalitarian and caring society at local, national and global levels. It sees health-care systems as first and foremost social institutions with power shifted to the critically informed community. It argues for a much stronger form of democracy, with genuine participation by citizens *qua* citizens in decision making around the social determinants of health. It puts forward a way of using this approach – communitarian claims – to empower citizens in a way that goes beyond rhetoric.

There are already examples of societies where these principles are applied successfully. Three examples are presented in Part V – Kerala (Chapter 15), Cuba (Chapter 16) and Venezuela (Chapter 17). All are community-focused. All involve citizen engagement and participation. All have eschewed neoliberalism. All succeed in terms of delivering good health to their populations.

The book finishes on a positive note. I believe that, particularly with the advent of global warming, there is a growing recognition that a new political economy is needed and that the planet cannot survive if we continue on the neoliberal growth path. One possible solution is presented in this book. What we need is debate about that and other options so that we can become a much healthier global community.

PART II

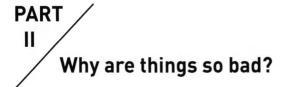

Why are things so bad?

1

Why has the economics of health-care policy gone wrong?

First, it is important to question who makes decisions about health-care policy both within and outside the system, and expose the influence of various actors, including the medical profession, the pharmaceutical industry, private health care and private health insurers. These are issues that come under the broad umbrella of the political economy of health care. They are too seldom discussed.

While there are many different definitions of political economy, that offered by Munro (2004: 146–7) is useful to our purposes here:

> a study of society and social processes. It focuses on 'material production' in two senses: (i) how the creation, distribution, exchange and consumption of goods, services, income and wealth occurs, and (ii) how the organisation and imperatives of material production influence almost all of society's other institutions, be they political, civil or cultural.

What I would add – just to be quite explicit – is that political economy is about power, specifically political power over resource allocation. Here the concern is about the political economy of health care; the next chapter is about the political economy of health; and the book as a whole is about the political economy of health and health care.

In health care, who decides – about what?

The question of 'Who decides?' in health care has to be followed by 'About what?' There are clinical issues with respect to patient care which are addressed by clinicians. There might at first sight seem little debate about the correctness of that. Yet such clinical decision making does not take place in a vacuum. There are budget limits; there may be restrictions placed on prescribing; the treatment of one patient may be affected by how many and what sorts of other patients the doctor or nurse is faced with, now or shortly. We know doctors are influenced by how they are paid. We thus need to be wary of thinking that 'clinical freedom' means unconstrained freedom to do whatever the clinical decision maker thinks is best for that patient, and accept also that doctors quite reasonably are influenced by what is good for themselves. In reality it turns out that there is substantial debate and disagreement about 'boundaries' to decision making here.

Where things get yet more interesting is at the planning and health-care policy level. Here there are multiple players: governments and politicians; managers, both lay and medical; the pharmaceutical industry; the private insurance sector; medical associations; nursing and other health-care professional associations; patients' associations; trade unions – the list can get very long. Some of these groups act within the system; others, even if seemingly operating from within, are outside influences.

One of the difficulties in discussing these issues lies in the notion that health, and as a result health care, quickly becomes 'everyone's business'. While one can defend that with respect to health, for health care it becomes more difficult. What is useful and potentially helpful is to look at the incentives or motivations for these different groups to be involved.

What emerges is that very few have an interest in health – population or individual – *for its own sake*. In saying that, I have no intent to deny the fact that many health-care professionals are most concerned with and about their patients' health, and in some cases I have no doubt this dominates (or even defines) their thinking. What is also striking is that few health-care professionals (except those in public health) have a concern for population health. Their focus when it is on health is on the individual patient's health, and rightly so. But can we expect that such a focus will maximise population health or lead to fairness in health or health-care resource allocation? That seems most unlikely.

For several of these listed groups, the prime interest is economic or more accurately financial, either through employment or profit.

As is exemplified in Chapter 10, the pharmaceutical industry is very clearly interested in profit maximisation and not in health maximisation. For some actors status matters. Managers and bureaucrats bring their own values to bear and press for more and better, for example, palliative care – forgetting they are there to serve the interests of the public in accordance with the values of the public.

There are so many 'vested interests' in and around health care. It is of note that in defining 'vested interests', the Collins dictionary, suggesting that it means 'you have a very strong reason for acting in a particular way', uses the examples of acting 'to protect your money, power, or reputation' – which is pretty close to the notion of status. All three of these interests are relevant for most of the groups listed above, but they are especially characteristic of medical associations.

Frighteningly, the question of who is to decide and about what in health care is too seldom asked, perhaps because those who currently hold power do not want the existing power structure challenged. The voice that is missing, that of the public, is unheard for two reasons. First, it is not wanted. Second, the public are too often confused between clinical decision making and other health-service decision making. Placing the medical profession on a pedestal for the first is fair enough; but in regard to the second such an attitude reveals a misunderstanding on the part of the public about the processes in question. It is also the case that the medical profession too often plays on the public's confusion, muddies the waters, and ends up with more power than is justified in health-service decision making.

Current political economy of health care

The discussion above is concerned with what might well be seen as the existing political economy of health care. How is this interpreted? Who better, surely, to inform the public on this than conventional health economists? So much of what passes for health economics today has been and remains dominated by the messages of Kenneth Arrow's classic 1963 piece on the nature of health care as a commodity (Arrow 1963). Health economists saw market failure in health care but really didn't know what to do about it. Indeed, this sub-discipline was slow to move far at all, concentrating on keeping as much of Arrow's paradigm as possible while embracing what essentially has become the medical model of the doctor–patient relationship: that is, a revised version of the principal–agent relationship, derived from conventional microeconomics. Bob Evans, the Canadian health economist, was one of the few who saw through this – first in his analysis of supplier-induced demand, but also, and more importantly, in his assessment of what lies behind medical practice variations (Evans 1990). He disputed the medical interpretation of what drives these variations – the Arrow-derived interpretation that focuses on uncertainty. Individual doctors don't know what good they are doing, so they all end up doing different things – hence variations. Evans argued that instead the problem arose because of *certainty*: each doctor was certain that what she or he was doing was the right thing! That is not only a fundamentally different interpretation; it leads to very different policy options – the former to better information on effectiveness to reduce doctors' uncertainty; and the latter to a big stick to get doctors to do what has been shown to be most efficient.

The attention that health economists have given to the Evans certainty hypothesis is all too limited, and Arrow's uncertainty altar remains virtually unopposed as the place for the true believers to worship. Thus Arrow has continued to set the tone for the political economy of health care.

The other major strand here, again taken from the medical model, is the idea that the demand for health care is a derived demand – that is, it is demanded not for its own sake but because there is a demand for health. That is fair enough, but historically the discussions then moved to an assumption (by health economists!) that the demand derived *exclusively* from health, thus not allowing that access *per se* to health care might be valued, along with, for example, being treated with dignity. That monopoly of health on the source of demand set the political economy of health care very firmly in the medical model. Since medicine is about health and really *only* health – at least if we look at what is measured in most clinical trials, most evidence-based medicine and clinical epidemiology – this served to confirm the place of the medical profession in the health-care power seat. Most conventional health economists abandoned cost–benefit analysis (which *inter alia* encompasses *all* benefits), to replace it with cost–utility analysis (which considers only health on the benefit side). That had two impacts on the power structure in health care. First, as indicated, it put the focus firmly on a single output which was very largely under the control of the medical profession; and, second, it pushed health economists into an exclusive focus on – perhaps an obsession with – health status measurement. We health economists believed we would have power and influence if only we could solve the riddle of measuring health – hence the obsession with 'Quality Adjusted Life Years' (QALYs) and QALY league tables. (QALYs are a measure of health status devised and used by health economists to bring together on one metric the two main health outputs of health-care systems – quantity of life and quality of life.)

There is nothing wrong with this as such. But what it has meant in practice is that health economists have neglected other areas. What about the decision-making processes? QALYs are strictly only valid (even in their own terms) if we are concerned to maximise QALYs using a form of marginal analysis where decisions on resource allocation are made on the basis of the ratio of marginal benefits (here measured in QALYs) to marginal costs across different clinical areas or programmes being equated. (That means, in practice, looking to see whether moving $x from heart disease to cancer treatment results in a 'better buy' in terms of whatever benefits we seek to produce.) The extent to which the health economist fraternity concerned itself with this issue (essentially priority setting) was, however, very limited, beyond a short period of fascination with QALY league tables, and a few who looked at programme budgeting and marginal analysis.

In other words, the setting for evaluation was sadly neglected, and that setting is in effect the political economy of health care. It was never seriously examined whether the political economy of health care needed to be challenged. As a result, two things happened: the power and influence of the medical profession remained much as before, and the power and influence of health economists remained much as before. (I am not arguing for the advancement of health economists as decision makers, but, used well, I think our techniques and ways of thinking can improve decision making around resource allocation.)

While there was a belief that health economists could measure health and in turn the Holy Grail of efficiency would be within our reach, that belief did not extend readily to resolving equity issues. This was reflected in an editorial in *Health Economics* in 1993 in which the late UK health economist Alan Williams (1993) urged economists to get to grips with equity given our relative failure do so until then. Looking back over the last 40 or 50 years of health economics, despite a number of excellent analyses of equity, the actual impact on resource allocation in health care to boost those regions which are deprived, or to discriminate positively in favour of the poor, has been all too limited. And why? We can speculate, but if the power base of health-care decision making does not shift, how can we expect any major movement of resources away from the haves to the have-nots? And if we do not recognise the nature of the political economy of health care and seek to change it, why should we be surprised if little changes on the ground?

Health care has been commodified and seen almost solely in the context of the treatment for an individual. The second level, where the concern is with the health-care system as a social institution, is largely ignored. In this sense, the framework of the market has been retained and there has been little or no recognition of wider considerations and value systems which might accommodate the idea of health care as a social institution – where not only outcomes are valued, but processes might also count.

There seems to be little in the health economics literature about a political economy of health care, which might include some of these broader considerations. Mackintosh and Koivusalo (2005: 6), however, in their political economy of health services, argue that 'health services must aim for universality of access according to need, and solidarity in provision and financing, and ... health systems should be judged against these objectives. Solidarity here is about robust redistribution and cross-subsidy to sustain access on the basis of need.' They add: 'This implies that health system performance should not be exclusively defined in terms of health outcomes.' Such thinking is most unusual, but also most welcome.

More observations on current health-care economics

There needs to be much more analysis of the power structures within health care, which is what much of this book is about. This is not to say that currently there is no political economy of health care. It is simply not possible to have a health-care system which operates in some sort of vacuum. What is needed is more detailed analysis of the existing political economy, an assessment of its merits against some socially determined criteria, a judgement about what changes are needed, and an examination of what routes to follow that will allow the changes to occur.

Many countries have public health services which appear to provide universal and equitable access, and there is a sense in which these attributes are present in practice. The issue beyond that, however, is just what we mean by these words – universal and equitable access. Take Australia, where there is a social insurance system called Medicare, which claims to provide universal access. Its website states:

> Welcome to Medicare – Australia's universal health-care system. Medicare ensures that all Australians have access to free or low-cost medical, optometrical and hospital care while being free to choose private health services and in special circumstances allied health services (www.medicareaustralia.gov.au/public/register/index.jsp).

The concept of universality gives the idea of a social service available to all, but not in the sense that television sets or bottles of beer are available to all. It also implies some notion of ease of access and in some, perhaps most instances, equality or equity of access. Often it seems to be argued that providing services at reduced fees or free (zero-priced) at the point of consumption will provide ease of access or even equality of access. Yet there are clearly other potential barriers which can be present and which can vary across different groups in the community: distance, culture and socio-economic status of the potential users. Distance is an obvious barrier and cultural barriers, for example for indigenous people, can be problematical. Socio-economic status can still be an influence even if fees are zero, as poor people are more likely to feel alienated by what are often middle-class staff in these services.

It follows from the above that the climate or socio-economic environment can be crucial. What that boils down to in many respects is the power structure or property rights over resource distribution: in other words, the political economy of health care. Particularly pertinent here is that branch of political economy known as 'institutional economics'.

What is meant by institutions in this context is rather different from or more extensive than the normal meaning. The view from Kasper and Streit (1998: 2) is helpful: 'Human interactions, including those in economic life, depend on some sort of trust which is based on an order that is facilitated by rules banning unpredictable and opportunistic behaviour. We call these rules "institutions". '

What is clear is that health economics has been obsessed with the micro, and often the very micro, and lost sight of institutional and macro issues. As Hodgson (2008: 251) argues: 'The predominant [health economics] mainstream focus in the literature has been on issues of measurement and quantification, to the relative neglect of the big questions.'

Hodgson draws attention to the oddity of health economists' views on neoclassical (essentially free-market) economics. He quotes Culyer (1991: ix), a leading UK health economist: 'In practice, the overwhelming majority of health economists use the familiar tools of neoclassical economics, though by no means all (possibly not even a majority) are committed to the welfarist (specifically the Paretian) approach usually adopted by mainstream neoclassicists when addressing normative issues.'

Hodgson responds: 'One is left wondering why neoclassical propositions are retained, when the standard normative apparatus of neoclassical theory is often abandoned. The adoption of some but not other elements in the standard neoclassical package is a bit odd' (Hodgson 2008: 237).

Hodgson is, I think, being deliberately polite and he himself goes on by implication to answer his own wondering. The problem here is that while we have, as health economists, seized on the fact that the market fails, we haven't quite persuaded ourselves to jettison all that rather wonderful (and also neat and tidy) neoclassical baggage with which so many of us grew up. We do not quite know where to go or where to turn. Certainly there is nothing around that is so beguilingly elegant nor so potentially measurable, and we have become such a quantified, seemingly 'rigorous' discipline that we cannot let go. At the same time as health economists have been beguiled, they have also neglected to build a new paradigm for their discipline, with the result that they have left the existing political economy of health care largely uncontested.

Another feature of this is at least as disturbing. This has played into the hands of the medical profession, who, with few exceptions, would want to encourage not necessarily private health care (although that would be true of many of their members) but certainly an unadulterated version of the doctor–patient relationship as being the cornerstone not only of clinical care but of health-care planning. The sanctity of that individualism is not only a crucial piece in the ethical base of medicine (fair enough) but it also protects the power base of the individual doctor and the profession. Challenging that power base, then, means also seeming to attack the individualistically based ethics of medicine – the ethics of virtue and the ethics of duty. Separating the criticism of the power base from the criticism of these individualistic ethics is crucial to the good planning of health care.

Good planning is vital but it is also based on another form of ethics – the ethics of the common good. That social ethic will inevitably clash with the medical ethics of virtue and duty. Thus while the concept of opportunity cost – the benefit forgone in the best alternative use of the resources – applies at all levels, for the clinician it is or should be restricted to the benefit forgone in the use of his or her resources on his or her patients. It should have no relevance to the dermatologist treating my skin problems what benefits are being forgone in delaying the treatment by Dr Jones of Jeannie Smith's hip replacement.

Conclusion

What this chapter identifies is that the economics of health care has suffered from treating health care all too much as a commodity and being seen by health economists and health policy makers as being very much the province of clinical medicine. This is in no way to deny the importance of clinical decision making and makers.

It is, however, to argue that clinical decision makers need to be restricted to clinical decision making.

These are issues that are best seen through the very neglected lens of political economy. They are also ethical issues, however, involving the clash of the individualistic ethics of medicine and the social ethics of health-care policy making and of what ought to be the ethics of health economics.

Some may be surprised at the lack of attention paid in this chapter to the power of the pharmaceutical industry. Some issues that might have arisen here are covered in Chapter 10. It is also the case that, while I have no desire to excuse the way in which that industry uses its very considerable power, a great deal of its bite is delivered through the medical profession. Take that route of influence away and Big Pharma would not be toothless – but it would certainly be bereft of its main incisors.

2 / Why have broader policies affecting health been inadequate?

It is quite remarkable in some ways that so little has happened – there are some exceptions – in the wake of the Report of the WHO Commission on Social Determinants of Health (SDH) (WHO 2008). There again, given the barriers faced by the Commission and the fact that acting on the SDH would be largely in the interests of the poor, perhaps it is not so surprising. The poor may be always with us. That prospect is more likely the less their voices are heard and the more societies become wrapped in the embrace of neoliberalism.

Shifting power

So many Western nations pride themselves on being democracies. Yet the extent to which that means that political and economic power is genuinely and equally in the hands of the people as a whole is all too limited. As we shall see in the example from South Africa, here is a country which set out, in the wake of the barbarism of apartheid, to arm itself with a very liberal constitution to ensure that it would never again fall foul of the power of minorities. Yet it has so sadly and badly failed. Neoliberalism has turned that democracy into a nightmare for the mass of the South African population; poverty remains endemic, and inequality is worse than in 1994.

We shall also see how Australia has failed to control the influence of the mining giants. Tax money that was needed to pay for more hospitals and other welfare benefits never materialised as the government succumbed to pressure from the mining industry.

In the UK in the wake of the bail-out of the big banks after the global financial crisis, there are massive cuts to public spending which are increasing poverty, income inequality and, very clearly, inequality of power. Indeed, we can readily argue that these are the result of the inequality in power. Further, they are resulting in serious concerns about the continuing viability of the NHS.

Globally there has been a diminution of the WHO's influence and a financialisation of policy on health and health care, as the IMF and, even more so, the World Bank have made their presence known in health policy globally. As Irwin and Scali (2005) write in a report for the SDH Commission:

> The late 1980s and early 1990s witnessed a waning of WHO's authority, with de facto leadership in global health seen to shift from WHO to the World Bank. In part this was a result of the Bank's vastly greater financial resources; by 1990, Bank lending in the population and health sector had surpassed WHO's total budget. In part the shift also reflected the Bank's elaboration of a comprehensive health policy framework that increasingly set the terms of international debate, even for its opponents.

The WHO's Commission on Social Determinants of Health

In all the gloom and doom surrounding the failure of so many governments and so many global institutions to embrace the social determinants of health, one beacon of hope appeared to be the WHO and its Commission on Social Determinants of Health (WHO 2008). This has done more to put the social determinants of health on the political and policy map than any other single event that I can think of. It has been taken up in principle in many quarters and by many governments. One has to try to be optimistic that it will make a difference in practice to population health.

And yet again, like its earlier companion report from the Commission on Macroeconomics and Health, it signally fails to get to grips with neoliberalism.

The sole reference by the authors to neoliberalism even merits being set in inverted commas! The full reference – and it is short – to issues around neoliberalism is as follows:

> Aspects of globalisation, such as trade liberalisation and market integration between countries, have brought major shifts in countries'

national productive and distributive policies. 'Structural adjustment' – a core global programmatic and policy influence from the 1970s onwards – framed the emergence of a dominant (sometimes referred to as 'neoliberal') orthodoxy in global institutions. Designed to reduce inflation in indebted developing countries, decrease public spending, and promote growth – all strongly oriented towards supporting debt repayment – adjustment policies promoted trade liberalisation, privatisation, and a reduced role for the public sector. This had a severe adverse impact on key social determinants of health – including health care and education – across most participating countries. Many countries, without doubt, stood to benefit from reducing runaway inflation and improving fiscal management. But it is not clear that the harsh degree and policy straitjacket that structural adjustment imposed produced the anticipated benefits, much less whether the health and social costs were warranted. (Jolly 1991)

That is it. There is a very substantial literature on neoliberalism and much written on its impact on health, yet the Commission decides it merits only one reference, and then an old article written by an insider from a UN organisation (UNICEF). The quote above is clearly critical of neoliberalism, suggesting that it had 'a severe adverse impact on key social determinants of health' but that criticism somehow disappears into thin air before we get to the recommendations of the report.

The report lists what it calls the 'structural drivers of health inequities' which highlights that 'the top fifth of the world's people in the richest countries enjoy 82 per cent of the expanding export trade', et cetera; that 'the East Asian financial crisis was triggered by a reversal of capital flows of around US$ 105 billion ... equivalent to 10 per cent of the combined gross domestic product (GDP) of the region'; 'since 1990, conflicts have directly killed 3.6 million people [and] many countries spend more on the military than on health'; 'each European cow attracts a subsidy of over US$2/day, greater than the daily income of half the world's population'. And so on.

Stunningly and disturbingly, there is no stepping back to show how neoliberalism has contributed to these problems. There is no structural analysis. It is as if the report has been sanitised to evade any attempt at structural analysis. The description of the problems is excellent; the analysis all too lacking. What an opportunity missed!

The state and the market

Let me turn to the role of the state in today's society and the fact that it is increasingly threatened by both globalisation and neoliberalism. The idea of the market is that it seeks to give each individual the right to define his or her own good on the basis that there is a right for everyone to choose whatever maximises that person's own good. This is freedom in classic liberal terms. But this is based on three premises that are too often skirted over by neoliberals. These are that choice involves the money or income to make such choices; that individuals' values and desires must coincide; and that socially the good is simply the sum of individual goods as defined by the individuals.

A related but separate issue here is that the neoclassical myth that money buys happiness and more money buys more happiness needs to be exposed together with the ideas from that same neoclassical school of economics of 'utility' and 'utility maximisation' for the distractions that they are. Maggiolini and Nanini (n.d.: 5) draw a distinction between utility and happiness, arguing that it is worth talking of two dimensions of well-being: 'the acquiring dimension – a person feels better if he/she has more goods, income and services'. This is the utility dimension. Then there is 'the expressive one that uses the way we establish relationships with other people', which is the happiness dimension. They sum this up neatly by adding (*ibid.*: 4): 'Even though utility can be maximised in solitude, happiness asks for two people, at least.'

More broadly and perhaps more significantly, the evidence to support the idea that money brings happiness is just not there. As Zarri (2006) remarks: 'Recent evidence suggests that money is less and less able to buy happiness and, in this light, Rabin (1993) correctly remarks that "Welfare economics should be concerned not only with the efficient allocation of material goods, but also with designing institutions such that people are happy about the way they interact with others".'

There is all too much emphasis on the developed world in the literature on the SDH. This is odd since the vast majority of health problems are in low- and middle-income countries. It is in the latter, too, that the social determinants of health matter most: there is often a lack of clean drinking water, poor housing and education, poverty and great inequality. It may be that the rich West's lack of political interest in the problems of developing countries is matched by a similar lack on the part of its academics and researchers.

With respect to a key social determinant of health – income inequality – however, there is all too little health economics research. It is significant that in the main reviews on inequalities in income and health by Wilkinson and Pickett (2006) and Deaton (2003), with 200 and 170 references respectively, there was no reference to any publication in the two major health economics journals. This neglect needs to be addressed.

The literature on health status measurement has a number of problems. Here, however, I want to draw attention to one that has not been given the attention it deserves. Questions surrounding culture and health, as in, for example, the destruction of Indigenous culture, have not often been seen as relevant territory for research. Yet it is clear that the relationship between land rights and Indigenous health, and the resource issues surrounding such matters, need detailed examination. More fundamentally, as Adams (2004: 283) indicates, 'Health is a product of social, economic, political, and religious social structures that are themselves shaped and constituted culturally and in contested political terrain.' Health economists have sought to deny or ignore this cultural issue and assumed that the construct of health is the same in all cultures. The idea that health might be constructed differently by different nations and different cultures is too often missing from discussions about health policy.

The literature on the political economy of the social determinants of health is sparse. Notable exceptions are several of the works of Bob Evans (1997, for example) and of Vicente Navarro (2007a); and coverage of the topics of road safety (see Jones-Lee 2002) and smoking (see Parrott and Godfrey 2008). There is little on housing, access to clean water, education and social structures more generally. It is quite remarkable how little there is on the key social determinants of inequality and poverty; almost nothing on the impact of the World Trade Organization (WTO) on world health; or on the effect of patenting regimes on income distribution between developed and developing worlds and thereby on health.

What research has been undertaken has been led by social epidemiologists like Marmot and Wilkinson. Certainly Vicente Navarro (2007a) and Angus Deaton (2003) have done some important work on inequalities and health, but overall there is a considerable lack of research on the political economy of the social determinants of health.

At the still broader level of social institutions and ideologies in a comparative international framework, looking at the WTO, for example, and the impact of its policies on health globally, political economy has been largely absent from the scene. The work of Navarro (2007a) and that of a few others such as Gwatkin (2001) are immediately noteworthy in terms of their quality, but also their rarity. David Coburn (2000), the Canadian sociologist, has made important contributions. The political economy of tax policy and its impact on health (except in goods taxes on alcohol and tobacco) through changes in income distribution are crying out to be analysed.

There has also been a neglect of how population health can be achieved and whether it necessarily need involve economic growth – though this issue is picked up by Sen (2001) in his comparison between growth-mediated and support-led progress. The former (*ibid.*: 338) 'works through fast economic growth and its success depends on the growth process being wide-based and economically broad ... and also on the utilisation of the enhanced economic prosperity to expand the relevant social services, including health care, education and social security. In contrast ... the 'support-led' process does not operate through fast economic growth but works through a programme of skilful social support of health care, education, and other relevant social arrangements.' Sen (*ibid.*: 338) quotes the examples of 'the experiences of economies such as Sri Lanka, pre-reform China, Costa Rica, or the Indian state of Kerala, which have had very rapid reductions in mortality rates and enhancement of living conditions, without much economic growth.'

A major problem with health policy is that it is too often dominated, even monopolised, by health-care policy. In turn, the latter frequently adopts a medical perspective. The distribution of property rights in health care results in the 'medicalisation' of this social institution and also of the health policy debate.

This medical perspective is also reflected in the approach that donors often adopt in giving aid to developing countries. Such giving is most frequently set along disease programme lines – targeting malaria, for example. What this means is that the emphasis is on investing in improving health outcomes directly. Too little attention is then given to building up the governance structure and relevant institutions to deliver good health care. The principle donors adopt in their aid giving then fail to reflect the wider perspective of the health-care system as a social institution, and do not take into account local values in deciding on investment strategies for health. Worse still, donors interested in health advancement seldom see beyond medical health care.

It is also the case that WHO and the World Bank tend to adopt a medical perspective. This is especially evident in the WHO's advocacy of the idea of the burden of disease for priority setting (see, for example, Murray and Lopez 1996). This is problematical at a number of levels. It sought to argue *inter alia* that the setting of priorities ought to be along disease lines. This is really rather peculiar because priority setting is only necessary because of the fact that resources are scarce. If this were not the case then choices and hence priorities would not be required. It is thus the situation that priorities must be about the use of resources, and it is interventions that use resources. It is interventions that need to be addressed and not diseases as such. Here again, however, it is the disease or medical model that WHO and the World Bank employ in this 'burden of disease' approach. The political economy analyses undertaken to ascertain why and how this might be changed are few and far between.

One of the problems for health policy is that when analysts and policy makers step outside the health-care sector, they quickly discover that the entities of population health and the social determinants of health are very big, very broad and somewhat amorphous. Measurement becomes more difficult as population health measures can include such intangible considerations as 'preparedness', which has been defined as follows:

> The capability of the public health and health-care systems, com-
> munities and individuals to prevent, protect against, quickly respond
> to and recover from health emergencies, particularly those whose scale,

timing or unpredictability threaten to overwhelm routine capabilities. Preparedness involves a coordinated and continuous process of planning and implementation that relies on measuring performance and taking corrective action. (RAND Corporation 2007)

Analysts are now on difficult ground; too often they want to focus on the measurable, which may well mean pulling back to measuring the outputs of the health-care system as other outputs are too daunting to measure. Going outside health care also means trying to embrace resources at the level of 'whole of government', as so many aspects of the social determinants of health fall outside the domain of health care. They can be slow to move to foreign territory and there can be a reluctance on the part of those in non-health-care silos, such as housing or the taxation office, to allow them in.

As I have indicated before (Mooney 2009),

A good example of some of these issues is the question of evidence-based policy which has become so prevalent in clinical medicine. While one might argue that the virtue of being evidence-based cannot be disputed, it is at the same time worrying that it has become something of a religion in clinical medicine (Kristiansen and Mooney 2004). One can see that evidence-based randomised controlled trials in evaluation of pharmaceuticals are both valuable and valid. Within clinical medicine however such evaluation in home care versus hospital care for sufferers from multiple sclerosis becomes more problematical. Extend the focus to evaluation of atmospheric pollutants or income inequality or Indigenous land rights and evidence is not just harder to come by but that which is required is of a very different type. It follows that the individualistic consequentialism of clinical evaluations is not only more difficult to apply to the social determinants of health but risks being described as attempting to 'weigh heat'. In the competition for resources for health, instead of the social determinants of health trying to compete with clinical medicine on the individualistic consequentialist paradigm of clinical medicine, it needs a separate paradigm. Otherwise it will continue to fail at that level.

The paradigm spelt out in Chapter 12 seeks to overcome this problem.

It is also likely that what different societies and different cultures characterise as the social determinants of health and their relative influences on population health will vary. Some will see clean water as crucial to survival; others, because they have it, will take it for granted. Some will place more weight on a healthy diet to avoid obesity; others on eating to avoid malnutrition. And all the time the construct of health has to be recognised as being to some extent culturally based.

Conclusion

What we currently have is too much emphasis on health care and not enough on health, particularly at a policy level; a reluctance on the part of governments in general, but with some notable exceptions, to get into the social determinants of health; a similar reluctance of health departments to step outside their comfort zone or to tread on the toes of their colleagues in other departments such as housing; a wariness on the part of researchers to move to this relatively new territory as it is not immediately clear what the outcomes are, or that they are measurable; a big gap in linking the social determinants of health to cultural issues and accepting that different cultures are likely to have different social determinants of health as well as different constructs of health; and, finally and perhaps most worrying of all, that even such an august body as the WHO Commission on Social Determinants of Health has a strange blindspot when it comes to getting beyond describing the problems that constitute the social determinants of health and setting out the symptoms. The failure of the Commission to do more than make mention of neoliberalism and its impact on health is astonishing.

Some governments, such as the UK and the European Commission, have been serious in trying to shift more of the emphasis in health policy from health care to health. Others, such as the Australian government, have dragged their feet. That needs to change.

The malaise of neoliberalism in health, health care and health economics

Neoliberalism

The birth of neoliberalism can be dated to the late 1970s and what became known as the 'Washington Consensus', although to what extent it constituted a consensus at all is doubtful. It was one man's assessment of 'what would be regarded in Washington as constituting a desirable set of economic policy reforms' (Williamson 2002). This was neoliberalism, an 'advanced' or more extreme form of capitalism which saw Keynesianism finally dead and buried. Indeed part of its role was to carry out that burial. Neoliberalism has been defined by Harvey (2005: 2) as 'a theory of political economic practices that proposes that human well-being can best be advanced by liberating individual entrepreneurial freedoms and skills within an institutional framework characterised by strong private property rights, free markets and free trade.... State interventions in markets ... must be kept to a bare minimum.' It is born of a belief in the market and its capacity to deliver efficiency in resource use in virtually all sectors of the economy and indeed of society more generally. It seemingly favours small government (but perhaps more accurately seeks minimum interference from government). In reality, as in the recent global financial crisis, neoliberals are willing to fall back on government, but on their terms. What has happened with neoliberalism as compared with earlier forms of capitalism is that increasingly the state has become corporatised. This inevitably threatens democracy.

We can note that nearly 70 years ago, Karl Polanyi forecast what Margaret Thatcher later infamously acknowledged ('there is no such thing as society') that 'to allow the market mechanism to be the sole director of the fate of human beings and their natural environment ... would result in the demolition of society' (Polanyi 1944: 76).

In more recent times Polanyi has been proved right, and Thatcher too, to the extent that rampant neoliberalism has resulted in what is a near-death experience for citizenship, society and the community. Most of us today in the 'liberal democratic' West have almost no role as citizens except to vote from time to time, and even then the influence of that voting is often heavily biased towards the rich and fortunate. As Galbraith (1996: 8) has argued: 'the modern political dialectic ... is an unequal contest: the rich and the comfortable have influence and money. And they vote. The concerned and the poor have numbers, but many of the poor, alas, do not vote. There is democracy, but in no slight measure is it the democracy of the fortunate.' As demonstrated in chapters 8 and 9, the corporatisation of government has reduced still further the influence of citizens on what their supposedly democratically elected governments do.

Neoliberals believe that the nature of the good society is based on the right of individuals to make their own choices to maximise their own individual good in whatever ways they want. Further they contend that this individual freedom is paramount. The good of the whole is simply a summation of the good of the individuals.

Harold Laski (1933), the British socialist of the mid-twentieth century, wrote of the impossibility of achieving the good society under capitalism. He argued that a good society could 'no more make peace between the motives of private profit and public service than it could continue to be half-slave and half-free' and went on to claim that '[t]he malaise of capitalist democracy was incurable while it remains capitalist' (*ibid.*: 164, 169).

I would suggest that, with respect to the social determinants of health, the major determinants are poverty and inequality. There is no doubt about poverty and that is intuitively clear. There is also now good evidence that inequality is bad for health (see, for example, Wilkinson and Pickett 2010). Where there remains some doubt is whose health is affected: potentially the whole unequal society or only those at the bottom. Being poor in an unequal society is worse for the health of the poor than it is for the poor in a more equal society. Thus being poor is bad; inequality makes it yet worse. Importantly in the context of this book, this is especially true if such inequality is set in terms of what Wilkinson and Pickett (2006) call 'social stratification or how hierarchical a society is', or what Navarro (2007b) calls class.

Whether the health of all groups is poorer is where the debate comes in. Quickly this becomes an ethical debate. Should we seek to reduce inequality because everyone's health is suffering (including the well-off, and if this is demonstrated they are more likely to support policies to reduce inequality) or because the health of the poor is suffering and the rich are prepared to pitch in to make things better for them? (The issue becomes much easier to handle if we adopt a more community-orientated perspective, as I will do later in the book.)

As I have argued previously (Mooney 2009: 92), 'There are various explanations for the impact of inequality on health but most relate to loss of autonomy and powerlessness. Being powerless is bad for health, as is being subjected to power. The greater the inequality in a society, the less cohesion and solidarity it has. Where societies lack compassion for the disadvantaged, inequalities are likely to be greater and likewise the impact of inequality on health. A class analysis such as Navarro advocates (2007b) is needed to allow a fuller understanding of the impact of inequality on health. This issue is thus to be seen not just in terms of inequality in income but inequality in power.'

In an earlier paper (Mooney 2005) I sought to examine the issue of addiction in the context of compassion, quoting Cohen (1997: 160) that 'the dominant opinion in the US seems to hold that the individuals who suffer ... conditions [of addiction] are the cause of them'. He suggests (*ibid.*: 161) that 'American politicians have neither the tools to fight the presence of growing masses of underclass poor nor the political support for creating such tools.' Drawing on that, I wrote (Mooney 2005: 140): 'Public compassion matters.... We need to care not simply because people who are poor in income or have had their culture destroyed by colonisation or are addicted to gambling or drugs, or have fled from some vile regime, but simply because they are badly off.... The need is to embrace rather than push away "the other".... To embrace must be for the sake of building a decent society, a caring community, for the sake of a common humanity, for community autonomy. The individualism of the market belongs to the market; it is not the basis for building a community or society.' It is this idea of building a decent society based on community values rather than the individualism that neoliberalism breeds that is crucial in thinking about reform.

This individualism is what the Canadian philosopher Charles Taylor (1991) calls *The Malaise of Modernity* in a book of the same title. He labels this 'the dark side of individualism' which centres 'on the self, which both flattens and narrows our lives, makes them poorer in meaning, and less concerned with others or society' (Taylor 1991: 4). I would argue that this malaise transfers to social, cultural and global concerns. It can flatten and narrow at these levels too, and thereby push for a monoculturalism across the globe. It can serve to make us inward-looking, failing to see the wider society and the benefits of being a member of it. In turn we can fail to see that our own cultures are being undermined as neoliberalism not only promises material reward but threatens social cohesion.

This malaise of modernity thus breeds uncaring societies and threatens societies with equally uncaring institutions. 'Flattened and narrowed' in our perspectives we become reduced to individuals – and society meanwhile first ceases to matter, then is faced with a risk of collapse. Those who see neoliberalism as some sort of pinnacle to human endeavour will find comfort 'in the smugness of Francis Fukuyama (1992) in *The End of History*, in which he argued that neoliberalism and the market represent the summit of social and political endeavour' (Mooney 2009).

To me social justice is central to public health. Yet with the growth of globalisation and neoliberalism over the last 30 years, social justice has suffered. Rich people get richer and rich countries get richer, and while there remains debate as to whether the poor are getting poorer, the gulf between rich and poor is increasing. It is evident that this has been exacerbated by neoliberal globalisation.

This was evidenced in the UNDP's *Human Development Report* of 1999 (UNDP 1999: 3):

> Inequality has been rising in many countries since the early 1980s. In China disparities are widening between the export-oriented regions

of the coast and the interior: the human poverty index is just under 20 per cent in coastal provinces, but more than 50 per cent in inland Guizhou. The countries of Eastern Europe and the CIS [the former Soviet Union] have registered some of the largest increases ever in the Gini coefficient, a measure of income inequality. OECD countries also registered big increases in inequality after the 1980s – especially Sweden, the United Kingdom and the United States.

A recent report from the OECD (2011) states that over the last two decades, income inequality has been increasing, with the top 10 per cent of households by income growing faster than the poorest in most OECD countries. It also records (*ibid.*: 6) that 'Inequality first began to rise in the late 1970s and early 1980s in some Anglophone countries, notably in the United Kingdom and the United States, followed by a more widespread increase from the late 1980s on.'

This timing and these locations are striking. It is generally considered that the birth of neoliberalism occurred in the late 1970s in the US and the UK, whence it then spread. The remedies suggested? 'Reforming tax and benefit policies is the most direct and powerful instrument to increase redistributive effects…. Government transfers – both in cash and in kind – have an important role to play to guarantee that low-income households do not fall further back in the income distribution' (*ibid.*: 12).

The problem with such 'direct and powerful' instruments is that to implement them would run totally counter to neoliberal thinking on low taxes and small government. So they tend not to happen. In the OECD countries generally over this period taxes have been falling and company taxes, for example, have dropped from an average of around 44 per cent to 31 per cent.

Being poor results in a loss of self-esteem. If the better-off seem not to care – and that is manifested in many different ways – then that loss of self-esteem is exacerbated. In a world of individualism fed by neoliberalism, how can we expect otherwise? And such loss of self-esteem, it has been shown, cannot be beneficial for health (Coburn 2000; Navarro 2002; Wilkinson 2005).

There is much evidence that the rich countries of the West do not care in any genuine way about the poor South. For example there is a UN target of 0.7 per cent of GNP for donor countries giving aid to the developing world. Few countries meet that derisory target. On average they give just 0.2–0.4 per cent, with only five OECD countries above 0.7 per cent (three of which are Scandinavian). The two countries at the bottom are Greece and the US with 0.16 and 0.17 per cent respectively.

Teaching on these issues recently in South Africa to students from all over sub-Saharan Africa, they struggled to understand how the West could be so mean, until there was a dawning of realisation as one remarked: 'The West just does not care.' There were then many heads nodding in agreement.

The West does not care, for example, that, with the freeing up of markets under neoliberal globalisation, by 'stealing' doctors and nurses from poor countries, they are creating very serious workforce shortages in these countries. This has been exposed by Maureen Mackintosh (2007) who writes of the perversities of such movement, with poor countries subsidising the training of health-care personnel for rich countries. As she explains (*ibid.*: 159), 'Migration from Africa to high-income countries ... worsens an already intolerable gulf. Its distributive effects may be measured by the perverse subsidy generated.' Yet in my own country of Australia, neither the government nor the health-care professional associations express any concern at this. Indeed at a World Conference of Medical Students' Associations in Australia, I was one of three invited speakers in a debate. The audience was made up of medical students from across the globe, many from developing countries and many with strong feelings about social justice. The other two speakers appealed to the students to come and work in Australia. These speakers were the then Minister for Health and the then President of the Australian Medical Association! There was no recognition until I spoke of the problems that would be created for the students' home countries if Australia did steal these doctors. (It is the only occasion in my whole career when I have received a standing ovation!)

This is an example of the selfishness of the neoliberal West and the lack of concern it has for developing countries' health. We do not care. We do not listen for the voices of the poor across the globe. If we listened we might hear and we might feel obliged to act. So, it is better not to listen. We can continue in Taylor's darkness of our individualism, shutting our minds to the suffering of the distant poor – and for most of the time they are distant. The solidarity that is needed, the humanity that is needed, is not there. While one cannot place the blame for that solely at the door of neoliberalism, there is no doubt in my mind that the sense of community that still existed in my youth and young adulthood is greatly diminished. Governments now talk of 'national interest', which means in practice selfish nationalistic interest, with overseas aid more and more driven not by humanitarian instincts but by the security of the nation – again in the 'national interest'. Social cohesion dies within countries and any sense of global cohesion with it. That situation might well be ameliorated if our international organisations – our global institutions – acted in the interests of the global community. They do not, as the next chapter shows.

Neoliberalism and health care

The key thing in looking at the question of private versus public in health care is to note the comment from Bob Evans (1997: 427) that this is not a debate about truly competitive markets 'but rather one managed by and for particular private interests'. He elaborates:

> [M]arket mechanisms yield distributional advantages for particular influential groups. (1) A more costly health-care system yields higher prices and incomes for suppliers – physicians, drug companies, and private insurers. (2) Private payment distributes overall system costs according to use (or expected use) of services, costing wealthier and healthier people less than finance from (income-related) taxation. (3) Wealthy and unhealthy people can purchase (real or perceived) better access or quality for themselves, without having to support a similar standard for others.

The issue then is really about power and the political economy of health care. The private market in health care, while being dressed up as the way to promote efficiency through competition, is driven not by that (although conceivably it might be a spin-off) but by powerful forces protecting both their own incomes and their own health. It is in the interests of the suppliers, primarily the doctors, to work in the more lucrative private sector, but also of the pharmaceutical industry to foster private health care, which is in general less regulated than the public sector and where higher prices are more obtainable. Finally it is in the interests of the rich to pay for their own health care and not have to pay through higher taxes for the health of the poor.

In this context it is relevant to note that there is a considerable economics literature on 'the commodity health care' to which back in time I have to confess I have contributed. There are a number of problems in 'commodifying' health care as if it were a truly marketable commodity. These lie in part with the assumed nature of what economists call 'the social welfare function' – which is what economists assume is to be maximised, with the resources available, in health care. This ends up after lengthy debate in the profession most often involving simply adding up individuals' utilities. Thus there is no allowance for what Sen (1977) calls commitment – the notion that one individual (A) might act towards another individual (B) in such a way that B's well-being is increased but A's decreased. This is what Sen calls 'counter preferential'. There is no thought of a community but only the individual. We are all free-floating atoms.

As is demonstrated later (Chapter 12) this problem can be overcome by considering the issue in terms of some community where the community itself is valued and what is to be maximised is not simply or purely the summation of the good of individuals *qua* individuals but the communal good. It is this concept of a common project that is missing from the analysis of health care as a commodity.

Another oddity in considering health care as a commodity is that in recent years there has been a move under what is called 'cost utility analysis' to narrow the outputs of health care to health only. Of course I am not disputing that health is the key output of health services – but is it the only one?

The derivation of this idea can be traced back to the English health economist Tony Culyer (1988). He suggested various possible objectives for health services: 'to maximise freedom of choice in sickness, to maximise utility, to maximise consumers' sovereignty'. He saw benefit (*ibid.*: 34) 'in choosing an objective that is ... likely to command a consensus, which is not particularly quirky nor merely the idiosyncratic view of a particular pressure group or the tenet of a major but controversial political and social ideology' (*ibid.*: 34). He concluded that the objective 'health services exist to promote health' is likely to 'command a consensus' and came up with the following goal for health-care services (*ibid.*: 35): 'given the resources available to the health services, the health of the community should be maximised'.

What this means is that many health economics analyses simply assume that we can see whether the effectiveness of health services is improving or not by establishing if health is expanding. In turn of course this can only be done if we can measure health and hence the massive investment in measuring health by health economists using 'quality adjusted life years' or 'QALYs'.

This thinking and strategy can be attributed partly to the commodification of health care. (I was asked once: if health economists could not measure QALYs, would this spell the end of health economics?) To some extent the approach may be understood as a function of a societal obsession (ever more pronounced since the latter part of the twentieth century) with measurement and quantification.

What all of this market-orientated thinking misses is that health-care systems are social institutions with potentially wider concerns that cannot be encapsulated in market commodities – caring, being cared for, wanting to build a decent society, fairness and so on. It does not attempt to find out what the community view is.

These issues – what the good is of health care, and who is to define it – form the basis of the critique of health-care economics in this book. Methodologically too, this is where the real challenge lies. Further, the issue of valuation becomes difficult when we are dealing with individuals who in many health-care situations are able to desire only inadequately (Sen 1992). The concern here is that desires and values become separate. This can happen for example for individuals who are poor or deprived, and who may previously have in some way sought to improve their lot (or follow their desires) and been thwarted or knocked back. If this thwarting is repeated, this can result in a truncating of desires. Such people may cease to aspire to achieve, in this case better health.

In a society which is not compassionate, which is individualistic, which worships at the altar of neoliberalism and where economic inequality is rife, it is much more likely that social mores will exhibit a lack of concern for the health of the poor and disadvantaged, and in such a society private sector health care is likely to be dominant. Societies with greater social solidarity – where neoliberalism is absent or less dominant, and there is greater egalitarianism – will tend to emphasise public health care more.

I have argued previously that one measure (accepting that it is far from perfect) of a society's public compassion is the size of its tax take, as this is an approximation of its collective willingness to 'sort out' the distributions that emerge in resource allocations, primarily incomes, in the rest of the economy. If we then look across the OECD countries at the size of the overall tax take, we find at the top Denmark and Sweden and at the bottom Mexico and Turkey (with the US fifth from the bottom). That listing of countries does not prove my point but I feel it suggests that some sort of index of public compassion along these lines might well be possible.

4 / Neoliberalism, the global institutions and health

Introduction

In the context of health it would immediately seem that the WHO is the main global organisation to be considered. However, as we shall see, WHO is actually relatively less important in world health than other global institutions such as the financial and trade organisations of the IMF, the World Bank and the WTO. Health is not their prime responsibility but their policies can and do have serious consequences for health – which they often fail to see.

A notable omission from that list of global institutions is the UN. I think it is sadly right to omit the UN and will shortly explain why. The relative 'absence' of the UN has a direct bearing on the global political economy and the way that is managed by our global institutions.

The World Health Organization

There is a tendency for global institutions to adopt a Western and often neoliberal perspective in viewing the world. The following example of the WHO is a case in point.

The WHO (2000) report on world health was built on what WHO considered to be the key factors for judging how good a health-care system was. On the basis of these, WHO created a world league table. The factors included such considerations as overall population health, responsiveness, access and equity.

With respect to equity, the WHO adopted a universalist position: its relative value as compared with other health-care objectives was assumed to be the same in all countries. There was no recognition that how the Irish and the Indians define and value health, equity or health care might differ. The WHO used its criteria and its weights and measures to form their judgements about the goodness and badness of a health-care system. This is increasingly common practice in global institutions, who seek to impose universalist (and almost always Western) values.

In its Commission on Macroeconomics and Health (CMH), the WHO sought to avoid upsetting the prevailing global political economy. The Commission argued that there are

> many reasons for the increased burden of disease on the poor. First, the poor are much more susceptible to disease because of lack of access to clean water and sanitation, safe housing, medical care, information about preventative behaviors, and adequate nutrition. Second, the poor are much less likely to seek medical care even when it is urgently needed.... Third ... out of pocket outlays for serious illness can push them into a poverty trap from which they do not recover. (WHO 2001: 23)

This is a description of the problems, not an analysis. It does not examine the global political economy that has brought these circumstances about. It appears ideologically neutral. The CMH, as Katz (2007) argues, 'reflects one particular economic perspective to the exclusion of all others'.

Why? It might be argued that the answer lies in two words: Jeffrey Sachs. Prior to being appointed as chair of the CMH, Sachs had an international record of not just believing in the market but, where he had been allowed to, actively promoting neoliberal policies. What happened in the old Soviet Union after the wall came down is a case in point (for this and other examples see Klein 2007).

All of that was known by those at WHO who appointed Sachs. It can only be concluded they wanted a report that did not rock the boat.

The World Trade Organization

The concerns of the WTO can be summarised as follows:

> 1. To assist in the free flow of trade by facilitating the removal of trade tariffs or other border restrictions on the import and export of goods and services.

2. To serve as a forum for trade negotiations; and

3. To settle trade disputes based upon an agreed legal foundation. (Ranson *et al.* 2002: 19)

Let me focus here on one particularly relevant aspect of the operations of the WTO. This is the TRIPS Agreement – the Agreement on Trade-Related Aspects of Intellectual Property Rights. Its aims are 'promotion of technological innovation; transfer and dissemination of technology; and contribution to the mutual advantage of producers and users of technological knowledge in a manner conducive to social and economic welfare' (Ranson *et al.* 2002: 22).

Yet Joseph Stiglitz, a former senior vice-president and chief economist of the World Bank, argued that 'TRIPS reflected the triumph of corporate interests in the United States and Europe over the broader interests of billions of people in the developing world. It was another instance in which more weight was given to profits than to other basic values – like the environment, or life itself' (2003: 105). Under a neoliberal WTO we cannot expect anything else.

If TRIPS were acting 'in a manner conducive to social and economic welfare', it would be having a much greater impact on the health of the poor across the globe than is the case, particularly through pharmaceuticals and vaccines for which TRIPS is in a position, if the WTO so chose, to make major differences. Yet it does not. For example the UNDP (1999) indicates that while three quarters of the world's population live in the Third World (and bear a yet higher percentage of the world's burden of disease), they consume only 14 per cent of global pharmaceuticals. Only a small minority, just over 1 per cent, of new medicines in the two decades up to 1997 were for tropical diseases (Pecoul *et al.* 1999); only 13 were applicable to tropical diseases. Ranson *et al.* (2002: 29) report: 'Developed countries currently hold 97 per cent of all patents world-wide; more than 80 per cent of the patents that have been granted in developing countries also belong to residents of developed countries.'

These sorts of figures are not unexpected. The WTO is primarily concerned with economics and finance – neoliberal economics and finance – and not health. There is not much of a market among the poor, so that in neoliberal terms there is little or no case for economic development. There is little scope for the poor to exercise choice, except of course as can be the case if they choose to fall into debt and borrow. Things will simply not get better through trade as long as the world governing body, the WTO, operates according to the dictates of the neoliberal market.

The situation with malaria, which is a massive global health problem, is instructive – as can be seen in the following comments by Rob Ridley, the WHO's Director of Tropical Disease Research (TDR):

> New drugs [for malaria] have come out at the rate of about two per decade. However, the level of investment that has produced that rate has now dropped off, due to the competitive nature of the pharmaceutical industry, and you essentially have the situation that malaria is a neglected disease. The industry is not competitively engaged, you have a disease for which there is a medical need but there is no competitive industrial R & D. The reasons for that are quite obvious. You look at the anti-bacterials market, that's about a 16 billion dollar market, and you get 3 new products a year, and in 1996 there were 92 antibacterials listed in the American Drug Index. Now, even with that level of activity, people are still worried about antibacterial drug resistance. With malaria, the market is a couple of hundred million [dollars], you're getting one to two products per decade, and many of those drugs are not affordable to Africans and are limited to travellers. From the industry perspective, R & D costs are very high, and the malaria market won't support the level of revenues needed to recapture expenses before patent expiry. (Ridley 2001)

So, in essence, if there is no market – in the sense that the sufferers, their insurance companies, and their governments have neither the willingness nor the ability to pay for drugs – then where is the pay-off from saving the poor from malaria? Drug companies are not in the business of charity or compassion. They seek to maximise their profits. Helping the poor is not good business. And let me be clear. I would ideally want the pharmaceutical industries to be caring organisations, but while the global rules set by the WTO are neoliberal rules, and while we all stand back and let this happen, why blame the companies who are playing by the rules? The problem is the neoliberal rules.

The WTO did at an earlier time seek to reduce world poverty. If it had been successful, this would clearly have been very beneficial to world health. This was the WTO's Doha Agreement on world trade, which since it was first set out in 2001 has been changed, weakened and virtually destroyed. In its original form it was stated that:

> We recognise the particular vulnerability of the least-developed countries and the special structural difficulties they face in the global economy. We are committed to addressing the marginalisation of least-developed countries in international trade and to improving their effective participation in the multilateral trading system. (WTO 2001)

A fine sentiment but essentially, as it turned out, empty words.

What is the likely impact of the Doha Agreement as it now stands, some ten years later? Various assessments have been made for a range of countries of the impact of the Agreement if it were to be implemented in full (Hertel and Winters 2006). Some countries were predicted to benefit. For example Emini *et al.* suggest for Cameroon that the Doha agreement is 'likely to relieve poverty mildly ... with falls in both overall poverty and income inequality, allowing 22,000 people to escape from poverty in net terms' (2006: 371). In the Philippines, however, it is likely to 'slightly increase poverty ... especially in rural areas and among the unemployed, self-employed, and rural low-educated' (Cororaton *et al.* 2006: 401).

In total it is apparent that there is much uncertainty as to whether the impact would be positive or negative. Even if implemented in full, the evidence suggests that its impact would be small. Hertel and Winters (2006: 28) argue that only if the Doha targets were to be 'ambitious', would they have a 'measurable impact ... on poverty'.

Such 'far-reaching' reform does not happen because the Western neoliberal societies do not want it. Somewhat tragically, Anderson *et al.* (2006: 521) estimate that 'the overall gains from a WTO accord could amount to US$96 billion, of which US$80 billion would be reaped by rich countries'!

Again, should we be surprised? Stiglitz (2003: 131) thinks not: 'Trade negotiators have little incentive to think about the environment, health matters or even the overall progress of science'.

At the time of writing (August 2011) it had just been announced that the 'Doha round of negotiations on world trade faces collapse unless world leaders can reach a final agreement to lift trade tariffs before the end of the year' (MercoPress 2011). This report is the death knell of the Doha Agreement. The chairs of the committee suggested that what was needed to break the deadlock was 'relatively small in size and involved limited political pain' (*ibid.*). Against a background of ten years of negotiation, the economic climate of the current post-Global Financial Crisis, and the fact that we have been here before (in 2008), there are no grounds whatsoever for believing that the powerful nations of the world will suddenly be prepared to accept even 'limited political pain'.

Indeed the reaction from Via Campesina (2008), the South American social justice group, on the 2008 collapse suggests we should have buried Doha then:

> In Geneva the talks collapsed on a very big and fundamental issue, the protection of the livelihoods of billions of peasants worldwide against the aggressive pressure by the USA and the EU to open markets for more food dumping by their multinationals. The ongoing pressures through WTO to destroy peasant based productions shows that the WTO should get out of agriculture!
>
> Given this deadlock, Via Campesina urges the governments not to waste time and resources to find compromises to finalise the Doha Round any more. The food and climate crisis needs solutions and policies defined outside the neoliberal free market model, outside the WTO framework. Policies based on the spirit of social justice and solidarity beyond the destructive corporate-based thinking of competition and pillage of resources.

Operating under the edicts of neoliberalism, the WTO negotiators were never ever going to agree to a package that would genuinely have helped the poor of the planet, or their health.

The World Bank

The major roles of the World Bank are to promote the economic development of the world's poorer countries and to assist developing countries through long-term financing of development projects and programmes, with an emphasis on private development. The distinctions between the IMF and the World Bank have diminished over time and the two organisations very often work in concert. Certainly with respect to structural adjustment programmes, there is nothing between them in their adoption of such strategies for providing loans to countries in financial trouble.

In 2010, voting within the World Bank was changed to increase the voice of developing countries, notably China. It is noteworthy, however, that prior to this the US had a disproportionately large share of the vote at just under 16 per cent. After the change, it still had a disproportionately large share of the vote – at just under 16 per cent!

Where, in the context of health, the two organisations perhaps differ most is that, since its report *Investing in Health* (World Bank 1993), the Bank has taken a much more active role in matters related to health and health care. In doing so the Bank, to a considerable extent, has sidelined the WHO. The latter is not well placed to follow up its ideas and policies with finance and funding to support them, whereas the World Bank is and has done so.

For example, it was World Bank thinking that shifted the whole debate on priority setting in health to what became known as the 'burden of disease' (as discussed briefly in Chapter 2). What this did was to argue that priorities should be determined primarily by the size of the problem. Diseases were ranked in terms of importance by how big a burden they created. WHO worked out priorities on a global basis using this 'BOD' methodology. That in itself is relatively harmless, if misguided, but more importantly the World Bank foisted this approach on individual countries, especially developing countries. That desire to standardise from on high is problematical on two fronts. First, it takes local autonomy away at the individual country level, and second it assumes that the measures of health adopted in measuring the burden of disease are universal.

The approach suffers from a number of other problems, but two in particular. First, it is disease-focused, and second it is a flawed strategy. The disease focus results in the concerns and thinking being about individual diseases only, with less attention than is needed to issues of governance and management, and in turn to health-care systems. Yet if progress is to be made a major vehicle will be health-care systems. For priority setting and planning, the issue is not the relative size of the burden – malaria, say, versus cancer – but what can be done about these problems given scarce resources and, often, poor health-service governance. In other words, it is about the political economy of health and health care – something with which the burden-of-disease approach signally fails to grapple.

The World Bank and the IMF are basically monocultural, which means Western in outlook. They are driven by neoliberal thinking. The background situation on the world stage is summed up by Marmot: 'So far, the benefits of globalisation have been largely asymmetrical, creating among countries and within populations winners and losers, with knock-on effects on health' (2006: 1160). The role the World Bank has played in this is substantial as it has fostered this form of globalisation, based inter alia on trade liberalisation.

It is of note that the 2009 report of the Independent Evaluation Group, an internal monitoring organisation of the World Bank, was highly critical of the impact of the World Bank's Health and Nutrition Group's support to low- and middle-income countries between 1997 and 2007 (Independent Evaluation Group 2009). Over that decade, US$17 billion was provided in country-level support to governments. Yet of the World Bank's health and nutrition programmes only two thirds had satisfactory out-comes and only 13 per cent of projects focused on the health of the poor.

The report recommended that the World Bank needed to '[b]etter define the efficiency objectives of its support and how efficiency will be improved and monitored .... Support improved health information systems and more frequent and vigorous evaluation of reforms' (ibid.: xxi). There is nothing about the failures of the underlying neoliberal thinking of the Bank – just 'more of the same but try harder'. There is nothing about the need to reflect different cultures with greater empathy and to make the Bank's policies more representative and more accountable to the people they seemingly seek to help.

The IMF

In considering these organisations it is necessary to set them in a historical context, tracing them back to the Bretton Woods Agreement of 1944 (Bretton Woods 1946) which was about setting up a new international monetary system. This created the International Monetary Fund (IMF) and the International Bank for Reconstruction and Development, later the World Bank. The IMF gives loans or guarantee credits to the member countries and provides money for projects such as roads and schools. It also provides loans through its so-called 'structural adjustment programmes' (SAPs) to assist countries to restructure their economies when they are in difficulty. The IMF loans are more usually given when there are short-term balance of payments problems. Such loans are again dependent on countries agreeing to certain reforms of their economies, which in practice means embracing neoliberalism.

What has emerged over time is a split in the power of the global institutions. In effect, 'the UN was not to be trusted with the "hard" instruments of development such as finance and macroeconomic policy making; that was to be the preserve of the Bretton Woods institutions [the IMF and the World Bank] with their system of weighted voting and firm control by the Western industrial countries' (Raffer and Singer 2001: 7). The UN is left with what Raffer and Singer describe as 'the "soft" instruments' which include 'food aid, technical assistance, children, women, social policy and, more recently, the environment'.

This split matters. The UN is based on one nation, one vote; the World Bank and the IMF on one dollar, one vote. What then follows is that the rich nations control the IMF and the World Bank and deny as best they can power to the UN, where the poorer nations have equal rights of voting. In turn what the UN might have controlled has been shifted to the G7 and the G8 – again, in other words, to the rich and powerful nations.

The IMF has seen some limited reforms. In 2009, the funds available for lending were increased from $250 billion to $750 billion. The voting rights were extended but were still heavily stacked in favour of the major nations of the West.

The operations of the World Bank and the IMF are highly relevant to any possible attack on poverty or on inequality – whether between North and South or within poor countries. International financial arrangements have been based on what are known as 'conditionalities'. These are conditions which are purportedly aimed at providing a country with the necessary ability to achieve short-term stability on which they might then 'grow the economy'. By the late 1980s the World Bank and the IMF had agreed that 'structural adjustment or economic reform packages were necessary to reduce distortions introduced by inappropriate government policies, eliminate structural rigidities, and permit the development of liberalised and more competitive markets' (Chakravarti 2005: 76). Thus conditionalities swiftly became neoliberal rules leading to what amounted to dictating to borrowers how to run their economies along neoliberal lines. As Chakravarti argues: 'the programmes would bind the borrower to a set of conditionalities intended to bring about sustainable budget deficits, monetary discipline, competitive exchange rates, and a general liberalisation of the economy' – in other words, to neoliberal economic reforms (2005: 76).

Keynes, the British economist who was so influential in setting up the new economic world order after Bretton Woods, wanted a fund which would make money available to support this economic order and which would be massive – amounting to 50 per cent of the value of the world's annual imports. (He also opposed the idea of what became known as conditionalities.) This fund, even with its tripling in 2010, now amounts in value to only 6 per cent of global imports. As Raffer and Singer state, the diminution of this fund is 'a measure of the degree to which our vision of international economic management has shrunk' (2001: 3). The global 'beneficence' foreseen by Keynes has gone and neoliberal forces rule.

What is clear is that the World Bank and the IMF are well placed to make a difference to world poverty and inequality, which in turn could have a massive impact on world health. They do not do so – and why? Because they are run along neoliberal lines and poverty reduction, inequality reduction and ill-health reduction do not rate on the neoliberal scale. The voting may change a little; the money available may increase; and there may be some promised softening of the terms of loan agreements. It is still neoliberalism.

As something of a case study in the failure of the IMF, the study by Stuckler *et al.* (2011) is very relevant. This looked at the extent to which donor aid for health got into the health system. For my purposes it was particularly important that the study distinguished between this 'aid displacement' for countries which undertook a new borrowing programme from the IMF and those which did not. The period covered was the decade to 2006.

What is meant by 'displacement'? The background to the study helps to explain. Normally two reasons are offered for the slowness of development in low- and middle-income countries. One is that any funding is not enough to get a country out of a kind of 'poverty trap'. Some sort of 'quantum leap' is needed. The second is corruption – recipient governments siphon off money to other ends – so the intended purpose is not carried through. The hypothesis of Stuckler and colleagues is that 'World Bank and IMF macro-economic policies, which specifically advise governments to divert aid to reserves to cope with aid volatility and keep government spending low, could be causing displacement of health aid' (*ibid.*: 67).

Their study indicates that this is the case. For every dollar in aid to countries which was intended to boost health-care expenditure, only 37 cents ended up as increased health spending. What is more alarming still is that when they looked at non-IMF-borrowing countries and compared these with IMF-borrowing countries, using constant US dollars, the figure for the former countries was 67 cents while for the latter the figure was 1 cent (*ibid.*).

The authors also looked at the question of how this might affect the growth of health-care systems. They based their answer on the estimated growth for each extra $10 of donor funding. '[U]nder an IMF program, countries would be expected to increase health system spending overall by about $7, about $0.60 of which would come from donor funding. In countries not borrowing from the IMF, health systems would be expected to grow by about $18, about $5.05 of which would come from the additional donor funds' (*ibid.*: 71).

These results of course do not in any way rule out the possible influences of the other factors mentioned above – the 'poverty trap' and corruption – but they do add an important additional explanation. Given the magnitude of the problems to be addressed, it has never seemed to me that the amounts given in health aid have been up to it. Clearly now to discover that of these amounts little more than a third actually reach health systems makes these efforts even more puny. It is of great concern that when the IMF is involved aid cannot be doing any good in health systems because it doesn't get there. This is truly astonishing.

Conclusion

The WHO, the WTO, the IMF and the World Bank need to be seen first and foremost in terms of global political economy. They are controlled by the rich West and they then act in the interests of the rich West. In doing so they adopt and seek to impose on middle- and low-income countries neoliberal policies. The halcyon days for the financial institutions that Keynes foresaw at Bretton Woods have evaporated in the wake of the onslaught of neolberalism and its lack of concern for social and health issues, its efforts to impose this ideology, and its resulting disregard for the wishes of local peoples and local cultures. Its captive institutions have been single-minded or blinkered in imposing their values and their interests, in the interests of the West.

These global institutions need more readily to acknowledge that they are supposed to represent the world and not just the rich and powerful. They must also recognise that their imposition of neoliberal policies has failed to deliver health to the poor of the planet.

PART III

Case studies

5 / The US: the fear of 'socialised' health care

Public intellectuals discuss the reforms

In 2009 the *New York Times* published a series of short articles on US perceptions of socialism in the wake of the hysteria around the socialism of Obama's health-care reforms (The Editors 2009). Eight highly distinguished academics and others set out their views. I must emphasise that these are not (as far as I know and can guess) members of the Tea Party; they are neither uneducated nor ignorant persons. They include the editor of *The Nation*, various professors, a dean of a school of government, and a visiting scholar at a prestigious university.

There are some very reasoned comments on this issue but others left me initially amused at how silly they are. Yet these are from US opinion leaders. Why else would the *New York Times* get them to write for it? My initial amusement was at best misplaced.

The series was introduced with the following words. 'It seems that whatever President Obama talks about – whether it's overhauling health care or regulating Wall Street, or telling schoolchildren to study hard – his opponents have called him a socialist.... What does the word mean today, nearly 20 years after the fall of the Berlin Wall?'

Thus Steven Hayward from the American Enterprise Institute:

[I]f we step back for a moment and consider 'socialism' more broadly as a steep increase in political control of or intervention in the economy – whether it be through a revival of Keynesian-style stimulus and things like 'cash for clunkers' subsidies, or through a government semi-takeover of the health-care sector – then the charge [that Obama is a socialist] appears more salient.

Keynesianism equated with socialism? The health-care reforms 'a government semi-takeover of the health-care sector'?

Andrew Hartman, an associate professor at Illinois State University, quotes, seemingly favourably, Whittaker Chambers when that author in 1952 was criticising communism. 'What I hit [in aiming at communism] was the forces of that great socialist revolution, which, in the name of liberalism … has been inching its ice cap over the nation for two decades.' And Hartman adds: 'Many conservatives would argue Obama and universal health care are the latest such ice storms.'

So it appears that it is a 'socialist revolution' which is hiding behind a cloak of liberalism. And universal health care will ice over the US – and presumably its freedoms, its justice and its defences of what is otherwise the good society. It is not just the meaning of socialism that is getting mangled; liberalism is taking a bit of a bashing as well.

Charles Dunn, dean of the School of Government at Regent University, argues that in the US 'today people are fighting rising socialist intrusions'. He suggests: 'Democracy needs a healthy balance and a dynamic tension between [liberty and equality] to survive.' That seems fair enough. But he goes on: '[C]onservatives intently believe that President Obama's policy proposals, especially on health care, will irreparably alter that balance and inflict irreversible damage. They see the stakes in this battle as nothing less than a fight for the historic soul of America.'

Then we had Michael Steele, the chairman of the Republican Party, calling Obama's plan 'socialism' (CBS News 2009). Remarkable – and I had thought that Obama's health-care reforms were about what are relatively minor tweakings of access for the poor to better health care.

When I started to look at this issue, I had seriously wondered what lay behind this fear of socialism regarding Obama's health-care reforms. It just did not make sense. What becomes clear from the above is that it is not socialism itself that is feared but some ridiculous distortion of the concept that is being put about as socialism.

The reforms

What are the reforms anyway? Well, in terms of most other countries' health-care systems they really do not go very far at all. In saying that, however, I have to acknowledge that in terms of universality and equity the US is starting from a very low base. There are different estimates, but around 35 million Americans are not insured and the numbers that might well be classed as underinsured in comparison to their peers in, say, the UK or many west European countries probably amounts to anything up to 50 per cent of the population. It is hardly surprising, then, that extending care to all will increase costs!

There have been numerous attempts to reform the US health-care system, which is both extremely expensive and extremely inequitable. Obama has at least succeeded in making some progress when so many of his predecessors, at least Democratic predecessors – no Republican president as far as I can ascertain has even tried – have failed. Eventually, however, it seems that health-care reform will go ahead, as 'President Obama signed legislation on March 23, 2010, to overhaul the nation's health-care system and guarantee access to medical insurance for tens of millions of Americans' (*New York Times* 2011).

What is this about? 'The health-care law seeks to extend insurance to more than 30 million people by expanding Medicaid and providing federal subsidies to help lower- and middle-income Americans buy private coverage' (*New York Times* 2011).

Within this, what has been particularly controversial is the involvement of government in health care, although in reality it is not involvement that is the issue but *additional* involvement. The government is already heavily involved through Medicaid, which is by and large for the poor and disadvantaged, and is funded by both the federal and state governments, and through Medicare, which is for the elderly and is wholly federally funded.

One particular bone of contention politically and ideologically is the idea of the so-called 'individual mandate'. This requires that all Americans buy health coverage, or if they fail to do so they will be fined. This is a central feature of the funding arrangements: if it were not there, it is argued, the coverage of the 30 million

Americans currently uninsured would not be possible because 'insurers argue only by requiring healthy people to have policies can they afford to treat those with expensive chronic conditions' (*New York Times* 2011).

Because this issue is such a major sticking point, there has been some give from Obama, in that this requirement can be waived (but not until 2017) in individual states, but only if there is some other mechanism introduced to provide coverage of the uninsured without adding yet more to health-care costs (Stolberg and Sack 2011).

For most outsiders to the US it seems extraordinary that there is such antagonism to what most developed countries already have and have had for many years. The reforms are primarily about introducing greater equity and allowing the 15 per cent uninsured (but certainly a much higher percentage of the sick) to be covered for health care at an affordable cost. This is hardly revolutionary, but again I have to recognize that my comment is made from outside the US.

Whence cometh the opposition? Well, the American Medical Association is a major opponent. In an interview, Dr Nancy H. Nielsen, president of the American Medical Association, said that the AMA 'absolutely oppose government control of health-care decisions or mandatory physician participation in any insurance plan' (Pear 2009). The AMA firmly and resolutely believes in the market, although on what basis is not always clear. Mainly it seems to be because of a belief that costs will escalate if the poor are allowed to have access to care (which is likely to be the case – if more people are treated, other things being equal, costs are bound to rise!). There is also ideological opposition to the government 'interfering' in the market. It is difficult to find any concern on the part of the AMA with equity and the fact that, if costs do rise because the poor get access to care, that must be because currently they are not getting care. It is not a public health issue for the AMA; it is an economic issue in terms of costs and assumed efficiency.

An answer to the AMA's problem? It is interesting to me, as another economist, that we get the plainest one from Victor Fuchs, probably America's most eminent health economist. It is also interesting that it emerges in his new book (Fuchs 2011) – or more accurately an update of his classic *Who Shall Live?* (Fuchs 1974) – when he writes of the limitations not of medicine nor of the AMA but of economics.

Fuchs points to the fact that with respect to health care, some hard choices need to be made. And discussing such choices 'reveals some of the limits of economics in dealing with the most fundamental questions of health and medical care. These questions are ultimately ones of value: What value do we put on saving a life? On reducing pain? On relieving anxiety? How do these values change when the life at stake is a relative's? A neighbour's? A stranger's?'

Economics, he points out, 'can explain how market prices are determined, but not how basic values are formed; it can tell us the consequences of various alternatives, but it cannot make the choices for us. These limitations will be with us always, for economics can never replace morals or ethics.' Nor, I would add, can medicine – although I am sure many doctors would disagree, as they see themselves as the bastion of medical ethics and morality. It is odd, but seldom do doctors think through the nature of choice. Or it might be better to rephrase that, and argue that they seldom see the need for choice, or recognise the concept of opportunity cost.

Ethics and values

Medicine is very much focused on the individual and in turn so too is medical ethics. The ethics of virtue – of doing good – is the ethics of doing good to the individual patient. There is also the ethics of duty, again very much focused on the individual patient level: the doctor's prime duty is to his or her patient. The third leg of ethics at this level is the ethics of the common good, which is largely missing from medical ethics or at least clinical medicine, although it has to be present in public health medicine. Yet that is where economics is focused. That does not mean that I disagree with Fuchs in suggesting that there are limits to economics when it comes to morality and ethics and the question of values more generally. The point I would make is that if economists can accept that there are limitations to their discipline when it comes to ethics and morality, I am then suggesting that there are also limits and limitations to the discipline of medicine when it comes to ethics and morality, especially with respect to the ethics and morality of the common good.

This leaves open the question of whose values are to count, if not those of doctors and economists. The values of patients? In some instances, yes – but where we are concerned with the ethics of the common good, as has to be the case when dealing with health-care systems and principles and priorities, at that level patients *qua* patients will almost certainly (and rightly, I would submit) be much more interested in resource allocation that emphasizes the individual ethics of duty and virtue. And why not?

The values of politicians? Yes, but I fear that in so many countries (and certainly including the US) politicians seem incapable, even with democratic mandates, of standing up to the pressures from the medical profession and the pharmaceutical industry.

It is worth going back in time to the 1990s, when the same Victor Fuchs (1996), in an address to the American Economic Association Conference, reviewed the state of the art of health economics. He suggested (*ibid.*: 20) that health economists 'must pay more attention to values than we have in the past. Through skilful analysis of the interactions between values and the conclusions of positive research, we will be able to contribute more effectively to public policy debates.' Fuchs's point is endorsed by Uwe Reinhardt (1992: 315) when he writes that 'to begin an exploration of alternative proposals for the reform of our [US] health system without first setting forth explicitly, and very clearly, the social values to which the reformed system is likely to adhere strikes at least this author as patently inefficient; it is a waste of time.' And he goes on to ask, 'Would it not be more efficient to explore the relative efficiency of alternative proposals that do conform to widely shared social values?' His point suggests a large part of the reason why I advocate the use of some form of deliberative democracy: my favourite, as indicated in Chapter 12, is citizens' juries.

So to what extent is 'the market' the problem in US health care? Well, it is easy to say 100 per cent! But the issue is far wider than health care *per se*, and it is not even some rational assessment of the market. There is a very deep-seated belief in the market in the US and trying to assess why is not easy. It is somehow written into the soul of the American people. It is not new; it seems it has been there throughout most of American history. The founding fathers were strong on freedom and that freedom became expressed as the freedom of the market. Government interference was to be abhorred. That freedom has been worshipped with almost religious fervour; it is to some extent born of religion. The following is taken from the Faith, Family, Freedom Alliance website, which 'is an educational, grassroots-oriented, non-partisan ... non-profit organisation ... [which] believe[s] that the Judeo-Christian values this [US] nation was founded on need to be protected and maintained in order to ensure the future for generations of Americans.'

This particular article is headed 'The free market: cornerstone of a free society'. It quotes a Dan Griswold, Associate Director of Trade Policy Studies at the Cato Institute. That institute 'owes its name to Cato's Letters, a series of essays published in eighteenth century England that presented a vision of society free from excessive government power'. Griswold states: 'Economic liberalization provides a counterweight to governmental power and creates space for civil society. And by promoting faster growth, trade promotes political freedom indirectly by creating an economically independent and political aware middle class.'

The article sets the belief in the market in historical perspective 'in the founding of the United States'.

> When King George III attempted to tax the colonists at will, the monarch made two mistakes; he had not counted on the fact that a higher standard of living raises citizens' expectations across the board, and he was threatening their livelihoods. The colonists expected the political rights that accompanied citizenship in the British Empire – primarily, the right to bring their grievances before the government. This was not merely a stand on principle; the Americans wanted to protect what they had built from a rapacious government.

Seen in that light, it hardly seems coincidental that many of the Founders were middle-class land owners, and that the right to property was mentioned so prominently in the writing of the Constitution. The Founding Fathers understood that economic freedom establishes the existence of a private sphere in society. This is the hedge that limits government power, and provides the foundation for successive political rights.

It goes on to draw some contemporary conclusions:

The liberating power of capitalism is not merely a domestic policy; reliance on the triumph of economic freedom over tyranny was also the strategy that won the Cold War ... the US adopted the policy of containment, betting that the fragile and stunted Soviet economy would be unable to withstand the pressure. When the Politburo cracked and instituted the policies of *glasnost* and *perestroika*, the virus of free enterprise was introduced into the Soviet system. (Faith, Family, Freedom Alliance website, no date)

Conclusion

While this worshipping at the altar of the market and the rather silly attempts to frighten the horses by calling Obama a socialist and his health-care reforms socialised medicine can seem rather puerile, it is striking, as reported above, that these sentiments are not restricted to some right-wing rabble. There are senior academics who endorse these ideas.

The history of attempts to reform the US health-care system is strewn with failures and perhaps that is understandable. In a sense, like 'the war on terror' and the concomitant fight to defend liberty, the fight to defend the market (and not just the market for health care) is a war against anyone and anything that threatens the market. This in turn becomes almost synonymous with the fight to defend the US. While one can ridicule a war on 'terror' and likewise the defence of the freedom of the market against socialism, in the eyes (and hearts) of many Americans, including some of their public intellectuals, this is a very real struggle and a mighty cause worth fighting for. Ridiculing that is easy but counter-productive. Overcoming these irrational fears is the goal – and that is hard.

6 / The UK National Health Service and the market

Ever since the Conservative government of Margaret Thatcher came to power in 1979, the National Health Service (NHS) has to a greater or lesser extent been at risk from market forces. With the election of the coalition government of the Conservatives and the Liberal Democrats in 2010, the NHS is probably more at risk from such forces than ever before in the six decades of its history. This chapter looks behind current and proposed changes. Are these driven by a concern for the health of the population or equity considerations? Or are the reforms based on some reality or belief that there are major inefficiencies in the use of NHS resources? Or is this just another push from the marketeers to try to extend their power to new territories?

The formation of the NHS

The NHS came into being on 1 July 1948. In power at that time was the Atlee Labour government, which had unexpectedly taken the reins after the Second World War finished in 1945. Unexpectedly, because Churchill, the conservatives' leader, having led the country through the war, had not unreasonably anticipated that his Conservative Party would gain power. Instead the country turned to Labour. Why? There are clearly a number of reasons but the one most relevant to this book is that the war had created a sense of 'togetherness', of community, of a breaking down of the old order and a new confidence in the working classes that their time had come after all the sacrifices of war. There was a sense of belonging; a more communitarian society than perhaps ever before; a recognition that pulling together during wartime had worked for the nation and might work in peacetime as well.

In policy terms this took a number of forms – for example, the nationalisation of the mines – but the most relevant of these for this book was the creation of the National Health Service. This is often attributed to Lord Beveridge and his report (Beveridge 1942), but that report recommended what would have been a pale imitation of what actually emerged. The real architect and builder of the NHS was Nye Bevan, who argued for and got a scheme which involved 'the complete takeover ... into one national service ... of both voluntary and municipal hospitals' (Public Records Office 1945).

Bevan took on the medical establishment – and won! He is, as far as I can ascertain, one of the very few health ministers in history anywhere on the globe who both tried to do so and succeeded. The shift of power to the political stage and away from the medical profession was enormous.

Market reform

When Margaret Thatcher came to power in 1979, she linked with President Reagan in the US to push forward the neoliberal market efforts urged by the Washington Consensus. It was only later in her tenure (in the late 1980s), however, that she turned her attention to health care, bringing in the US economist Alain Enthoven (1985) to argue the case for greater competition in health care through what was known as the 'internal market'. This was essentially an attempt to bring market forces to bear without actually denationalising the NHS, although many believed that that was the road Thatcher wanted to go down.

Somewhat surprisingly to many, when the Labour Government and Tony Blair assumed power in 1997, there was less change than had been envisaged and certainly no return to the pre-Thatcher period. Thus, when in 2010 the Conservatives won power in a coalition with the Liberal Democrats, it might be argued that the die was cast (Lansley 2010). If more left-wing governments could at least partially go down the market road, the new government, which was quite openly and historically the party of the market, could be expected to go further, both ideologically and in policy terms, down the privatisation road. That is what is happening. At the time of writing (August 2011) the details of what will eventuate remain unclear and I will not pursue them. (For an excellent early account, see Hunter 2011.)

What I want to examine here is the source of the market thinking lying behind the changes, and the form it has taken. I thus want to look behind the statement made by David Hunter 'that the NHS in its current form may not survive the changes, as they open the way to privatisation and a weakening of its public sector ethos'. Hunter argues that reform after reform has failed and, while there is no single cause for these failures, the key issue seems to be that reform has been introduced without looking at the considerable evidence that exists on how to reform and how not to reform: this process – the failure to consult the evidence – he calls 'the triumph of hope over experience'. Hunter suggests that flaws in various efforts to reform the NHS have centred 'on the commitment to market-style policies embracing choice and competition where, at best, the evidence is equivocal that they will have the desired effect' (Hunter 2011: 166).

In the assessment of the internal market reforms of Thatcher's day, the general consensus seems to be that less change occurred than was anticipated. As so often seems to happen when market forces are let loose and the results do not live up to the hopes of the architects, instead of arguing that maybe the market forces were the problem, some argued that they did not go far enough. Thus for Le Grand, Mays and Dixon 'the incentives were weak and the constraints were too strong' (1998: 129).

While the Blair government, before its election victory, argued against market forces in the NHS, once in power 'there was a lack of conviction [to abandon market forces] and a perception emanating from both the Prime Minister, Tony Blair, and some of his special advisers, that a modernized NHS required some of the levers and incentives that had been a feature of the previous government's internal market changes' (Hunter 2011: 168). But again we must ask: why?

There is a simple explanation of the drive for reform, the ignoring of experience and evidence, and the lack of clear analysis in the case of the NHS. It is that all governments since Thatcher's have in reality believed in the neoliberal market. When they wanted to reform health, that almost fundamental belief came into play. If one is a believer, one does not have to have evidence or listen to experience or learn from history. The market will deliver. It does not need to be tested or evaluated. It is significant that Thatcher introduced her reforms in such a way and at such breakneck speed that it was not possible to get good 'before' data to allow a rigorous 'before and after' evaluation study design to be established. (The New Zealand market reforms were similarly introduced very hastily, at least in part for the same reason.) In a way I have some sympathy for the NHS reformers. Where else could they go for ideas for reform other than the market? There was Cuba (see Chapter 16) – but it would not look good to be copying a socialist country. There was Scandinavia – but their systems were rather similar to the NHS, so that would hardly constitute reform. Beyond that, no one else seemed to have much idea. The local UK health economists were saying very little about systems and were seemingly caught up in micro measurement issues around health. There was so little on the political economy of health and health care (with the important exception of the RAWP Report (DHSS 1976), which looked at geographical equity). So it was hardly surprising that Thatcher called in a US expert who then advocated market reforms – and that Blair, Brown and now Cameron follow suit. The ideas put forward in chapters 12, 13 and 14 were not around, at least not in that form, although Richard Titmuss's *The Gift Relationship* (1970) can be seen as a precursor of these ideas.

In effect, Titmuss's interpretation of the NHS was that it was 'very communitarian'. The problem was that that interpretation was wrong. He was right to see the altruism involved but it was an altruism that was imposed from above – and communitarianism, while in a sense based on altruism, is more about sharing and caring, reciprocity and mutuality. These characteristics cannot be imposed on a society.

What I am proposing is that the NHS be seen not so much as a national health service but as a series of local health services under the umbrella of an NHS. While that will lead to some tricky issues in terms of equity between different areas, there is no reason to believe that these cannot be overcome, for example through appropriate levels and arrangements for funding. The current UK government claims that the key focus of its reforms is local. That to me is a dubious claim. But the ideas in chapters 12 and 13 of tapping into local values and allowing critically informed citizens through citizens' juries to have their say in setting the principles that are to underpin 'their' health care would allow a genuine attempt to make health care local. That would not in itself be enough to overcome any obsession with market forces – but it might, in time, if the values of critically informed citizens were to become the basis of health-care planning.

Experience elsewhere

As something of an aside it is worth looking at what happened in Denmark and the way the Danes handled the issue of dealing with the threat or promise of more market forces. I believe the Danes found themselves on the whole quite happy with their very largely public health services. They were, however, aware that things were changing elsewhere and that market forces were being touted as the way to improve health services. A group of academics, on behalf of the Danish health-care system, therefore arranged to have a panel of 'experts' – one from each of the US, the UK, Sweden, the Netherlands and Australia – look at their health-care system and report on what they found. (I was the Australian 'expert'.)

The Danish health-care system is not perfect, but the overall assessment of the experts was 'steady as she goes', and that the system by and large is efficient, equitable and in tune with Danish values. We found no reason to argue for greater competition or more privatisation.

What is particularly interesting to me is that I would conjecture that the study was set up to show just that. I am not suggesting that the Danes are complacent about their health-care system, but they think it is pretty good – and they are right. They think it largely reflects local values (both Danish nationally and regionally within Denmark, perhaps not surprisingly as the services are run by the county councils). And they do not think that injecting market values will help to improve their health services, nor reflect better Danish values. But rather than appear complacent, they called in outside experts to tell them what they already knew – whom they could then quote!

Another country that has much more thoroughly reviewed its health services is Canada (Romanow 2002). I was involved in that in a small way with my colleague Alan Shiell (Shiell and Mooney 2002). We were asked to try to ascertain whether Canada could afford to continue its public health services. We argued very simply that it could if that was what the Canadian people wanted. That argument seemed to carry the day in the Commission's report, but again it is clear that the issue had to be addressed in Canada to fend off the privateers.

What is remarkable about the UK is that at no time have they stopped to carry out a review such as Romanow's, or such as the Danes commissioned, to establish, in any sort of detail, what the problems are with the NHS – and only thereafter see whether more market reliance would resolve these problems. But I suppose that if you have a fundamental belief in anything, such as the market, then there is no need to seek to test the rights and wrongs of the policy prescriptions that emerge from that deeply held belief.

The public sector ethos

Does it matter that the NHS retains its current public sector status and fights off marketisation? Is the belief in public provision and funding just as much an issue as the belief in the market? Is one more justified than the other?

One way to look at this is to examine the concern expressed in the quote above from Hunter about the possible weakening of the 'public sector ethos' which might follow from the current reforms to the NHS. It is then reasonable to ask two questions. What is this 'public sector ethos'? And what difference would it make if it were weakened?

To answer the first question let me go back to Nye Bevan (1952) the founder of the NHS. He argued:

> No society can legitimately call itself civilised if a sick person is denied medical aid because of lack of means…. Society becomes more wholesome, more serene, and spiritually healthier, if it knows that its citizens have at the back of their consciousness the knowledge that not

only themselves but all their fellows, have access, when ill, to the best that medical skill can provide.

The public sector ethos is primarily about fairness, of both funding and delivery. It is about seeking to provide care that is equally accessible to all, irrespective of income – with no greater financial barriers for the poor than for the rich. It is at the same time about building a culture within health services that recognises that for the individual health-care professional this accessibility issue means or even requires that a culture of non-discrimination rules.

Does it matter? That can only be answered subjectively. What is clear is that it is difficult to see how marketisation can deliver equity. Does that matter: does equity matter? That is a question that will almost certainly get varying responses depending on the country in which it is asked. Having said that, it does seem that in most countries some weight will be attached to equity in health care, but how equity is defined will vary, as will the weight attached to it.

Weakening the public sector ethos will make changes in how health care is delivered. Most fundamentally the aspect that will be weakened is equity. The market struggles to deliver equity. Efficiency is trickier. What can be said I believe is that what public and private seek to provide are different, so to some extent the argument is irresolvable. Efficiency comparisons are also difficult to measure because there is often also a difference in financing and, for example, a difference in how doctors are paid.

Such matters are to some degree cultural and may revolve around not only the outcomes of health care, such as improvements in health status, but also around how any society values its health-care system as an institution. Social institutions are likely to be valued differently by people in different societies depending on how they see them fitting into their conceptualisation of a 'decent society'. How that is interpreted will clearly vary from society to society!

A final word

Let me leave the last word with Alain Enthoven (2006), who many believe was the real architect of the market reforms of the NHS.

Writing in 2006 and reflecting back on his market reforms to the NHS from 1989 onwards, he notes: 'In 1998, I could find some evidence of improved economic performance, but not much, and not very strong. Important measures of outcomes, service and satisfaction were lacking.' His solution, however, was not to abandon market reforms but to argue that they hadn't been taken far enough!

7

South Africa, neoliberalism and HIV/AIDS

The impact of neoliberalism on health in South Africa has been devastating. This chapter examines certain aspects of this, first looking at HIV/AIDS but then at health more generally. (For a fuller account of health in South Africa see Coovadia *et al.* 2009.) The effects of HIV/AIDS on the population have been both serious and tragic. While policy here was long dominated by the irrational attitudes of President Thabo Mbeki and his health minister Tshabalala Msimang, the roles of the pharmaceutical corporations in failing to contain – and of the mining corporations in furthering – its spread have not been as well documented. Behind these, and at the more general level, have been the activities of the WTO and the World Bank.

HIV/AIDS and the pharmaceutical industry

An example of the workings of the WTO serves to illustrate the neoliberal focus of its power base. In 2002, in the wake of a well-publicised campaign, the South African government sought cheaper drugs from the pharmaceutical companies for their AIDS patients. The companies were forced by Amnesty International and public opinion more generally to back down and agree. At the WTO meeting in November 2002, it was announced that the WTO would allow cheaper drugs for developing countries (Mason 2003).

Then, a month later, the WTO changed its mind. They did so because the US pharmaceutical companies objected to the impact that cheaper drugs for South African AIDS victims would have had on their profits. As Mason (2003) writes, explaining the back-down: 'the pharmaceutical companies ... are determined to maintain their profits. The largest US drug company made $37 billion in profits [in 2001], a rate of return to shareholders of 39 per cent. Although less than 20 per cent of these profits are made from the 80 per cent of the world's population in the developing world, they are not prepared to allow cheap drug production to continue.' This is an example of neoliberalism at work at the WTO, in this instance through the power of the pharmaceutical companies. Fortunately the decision was reversed again later.

The way this affair has been interpreted is also revealing. Spritzler (2001) brings out the role of the economist Jeffrey Sachs. It was Sachs who famously argued that 'an economy can be reoriented from a dead end, a dead end of socialism or a dead end of mass corruption or a dead end of central planning, to a normal market economy' (quoted in Klein 2007: 145). He spoke at an AIDS conference in Chicago in February 2001, where he asked the US government to provide $2 billion to buy HIV drugs from pharmaceutical companies.

While agreeing that Sachs tapped into an important vein of concern that so many have expressed for the millions suffering from HIV/AIDS in sub-Saharan Africa, Spritzler described the speech as 'profoundly dishonest.' Sachs had stated: 'The essence of Africa's crisis is fundamentally its extreme poverty and therefore its inability to mobilize out of its own resources even the barest of minimum resources to address any of the public health crises that Africa faces.'

Spritzler suggests that Sachs is an apologist for the West and for neoliberalism. He quotes Sachs as saying: 'The international response [to the AIDS epidemic in Africa] essentially could not have been less ... a lot of hand-wringing but no real assistance .... We [the West] have essentially done nothing.'

That is all true in my assessment, but, as Spritzler goes on: 'An honest speech from a world-renowned economist would have explained how poverty and related conditions that are driving the AIDS epidemic in Africa are not the cause of Africa's problems, they are the symptoms of corporate exploitation of Africa; and any attempted solution which fails to deal with this reality cannot succeed.' It is that last comment that seems so important. Africa is not a poor continent; it is impoverished. Centuries of colonialism, of global economic 'rules' weighted against poor countries have taken their toll.

Spritzler argues in conclusion: 'in the short term, the pressure on political and corporate leaders to provide AIDS drugs to Africa will be greater if Jeffery Sachs fails in his efforts to divert criticism away from them, because their fear of being perceived as part of the problem instead of the solution is the only reason they have for providing the drugs in the first place'. That fear is driven by a concern over possible interference in their pursuit of the goals of the company. Being seen as bad guys is not good for business or profits.

Before leaving HIV/AIDS, it is important to recognise the impact of another industrial sector, beyond the pharmaceutical industry, on the epidemic, namely mining. Employment practices which separate families and the transience of the labour force in this sector have been identified as having a causal link to the spread of HIV/AIDS within South Africa (Epstein 2002) – and also beyond that country's borders, as many AIDS-afflicted foreign miners returned to impoverished communities in other Southern African countries, with no recourse to compensation or health care.

Mbeki and his health minister Tshabalala Msimang, in my view, were largely responsible for the epidemic getting out of hand; that is well documented. It could have been contained much more successfully, however, if the pharmaceutical industry, first, but also the mining industry had not been so hell-bent on profit seeking. With respect to the former, a different sort of WTO, one not driven by a neoliberal ideology, could have mandated the pharmaceutical industry to act more humanely.

At the WTO around this time there were ongoing discussions regarding exceptional provisions to ensure that patent protection for pharmaceutical products would not block poor countries from gaining access to medicines. According to Global Governance Watch (nd), however, some governments were 'unsure of how these would be interpreted, and how far their right to use them would be respected'.

As a result, in November 2001 the WTO came up with a Special Declaration on the TRIPS Agreement and Public Health (*ibid.*). In this, 'the WTO ministers agreed that the TRIPS Agreement does not and should not prevent members from taking measures to protect public health. They underscored the ability of countries to use the flexibilities that are built into the TRIPS Agreement, and they agreed to extend exemptions on pharmaceutical patent protection for least-developed countries until 2016.'

It is remarkable that these potentially fine words reflecting potentially fine policies to protect the health of people in developing countries came from the WTO, which then sold out on those suffering from and threatened by HIV/AIDS in South Africa. As reported above, in November 2002 the WTO stayed true to this sentiment to help the peoples of developing countries in pursuing better health by allowing cheaper drugs for developing countries. Then, a month later, they changed their minds under pressure from the US's 'Big Pharma'.

South African health care

Looking at South African health care, I want to go back to Nye Bevan's collective principle (Bevan 1952), previously quoted in Chapter 6, 'that no society can legitimately call itself civilized if a sick person is denied medical aid because of lack of means'. In South Africa the very latest figures (Department of Health 2011) show neoliberal policies at work. 'The 8.3 per cent of GDP spent on health is split as 4.1 per cent in the private sector and 4.2 per cent in the public sector. The 4.1 per cent spend covers 16.2 per cent of the population, (8.2 million people) who are largely on medical [private] schemes. The remaining 4.2 per cent is spent on 84 per cent of the population (42 million people) who mainly utilise the public health-care sector.' This is not only because the public sector is grossly underfunded and the private sector so large though for so few; it is also that the private sector is grossly inefficient, with over 120 medical aid schemes and sharply rising costs. Clearly, too, those in the private sector are on average healthier.

Thus in today's South Africa the split in health-care spending between public and private is unfair, no matter how one defines fairness. It is not in line with the South African constitution, which states that 'Everyone has the right to have access to (a) health care services, including reproductive health care; (b) sufficient food and water; and social security, including, if they are unable to support themselves and their dependants, appropriate social assistance.' Importantly, it adds that 'The state must take reasonable legislative and other measures, within its available resources, to achieve the progressive realisation of each of these rights.'

The current split between public and private cannot be efficient; it cannot be providing the most health benefit possible with the resources being expended. Thus the current service fails badly in terms of both efficiency and equity. Before the private sector in South Africa is allowed to wither on the vine there needs to be some more strategic political economy thinking. That starts with building up the public sector; creating a new management and governance structure; improving the quality of care in the public sector and the perception of the quality of that care. Then, and only then, should the private sector be thrown to the wolves. One advantage the British had when their NHS was founded was that there was no equivalent public sector in the UK as there is today in South Africa, so there was no benchmark regarding what the quality of care in the new NHS would be like. Unfortunately, South Africa currently has a public health-care system that functions very poorly, primarily as it is starved of resources. Additionally, the management processes are very bureaucratic; the management culture is demoralised and demoralising; and there is a perception that the quality of the public sector is low.

There is no need in the longer run for a private sector of any size. However, I accept in any transitional period that the death of the private sector at this point in South Africa's health-care system's history is in no one's interests. In making the case for the health service to be seen as a social institution, I will argue the moral and ethical case and indeed the socially just case for a public as compared to a private health-care system.

That situation arises from the existing power structure within health care and also the wider society; it is not about any rational economic analysis of priority setting. There needs to be a change in power structure – both within the health-care system and with respect to it. These changes cannot and will not occur without a change in the social and economic structure of South African society.

A National Health Insurance scheme is planned by the ANC government (Department of Health 2011), with an intent to pass legislation to introduce it in 2012, although it will take 14 years to be implemented in full. There have been wildly exaggerated estimates from the private sector as to how much such a scheme will cost.

The main opposition party in South Africa, the Democratic Alliance, has argued that the 'NHI will prove disastrous for South Africa', suggesting that 'both the quality of health care and the economy will suffer' (Democratic Alliance 2009). Part of its case is that 'the poor will be hardest hit, because the NHI does nothing to address the crisis in public health care.... The NHI is not pro-poor. In fact it is anti-poor. It is a sure-fire recipe for the destruction of public health care.'

The Democratic Alliance defends the private system as key to the future of health care: 'Quality health care in the private sector is available to a few, but at a high cost. The potential exists to bring these two sectors together to build a system that suits everyone's needs, and provides quality care to all.'

What are the choices and what might they cost in reality? Di McIntyre (2010) has set these out: 'The total resource requirements for the 'mandatory extension of medical scheme coverage' option (or SHI) are considerable. Only one country in the world has spending levels as high as 13 per cent of GDP – the USA. In my view, this option is unaffordable in the South African context. The basis for this conclusion is that the burden on households that are required to join a medical scheme will be very high, with scheme contribution rates per person being twice as high as they currently are in real terms.'

McIntyre (2010) argues that the main question is whether to keep the existing set-up or pursue a universal system. She estimates that

> the 'universal coverage' option would see health spending levels increasing in line with expected economic (GDP) growth, so that when fully implemented, total health-care spending as a percentage of GDP would be comparable to what it currently is. However, the key challenge with pursuing universal coverage is the need to allocate more public funds to the health sector, partly through increased taxation.

South African health

A class dialogue is seemingly absent in South Africa today. In the wake of apartheid, racial and ethnic divides are dominant, or perceived to be, so that class is seen as redundant or invisible.

If ill-health is to be addressed realistically, it must be through poverty reduction and inequality reduction. Yes, an NHI will help and that in itself can be redistributive. But it will not be enough. Jobs, houses and direct income redistribution are needed. Power redistribution is needed, and that means a class analysis. This is not to argue that being black in South Africa is not deleterious to one's health; it clearly is for most. But as the major power structures of white South Africa in apartheid times increasingly take on board the black elite, primarily to protect themselves, so the visibility of class becomes more evident. What is then needed is not just a bigger tax take and redistribution of money but, as important and almost certainly more so, of political power. I see no other way. Trickle down is a fantasy. The forces of neoliberalism in country after country defy the forces of gravity and instead we have trickle up. South Africa will not buck this trend.

The culprits for the persistence of poor health are poverty and inequality. Poverty has increased in the poorest households since 1994. Over the same time period income inequality has increased. And why? Because the ANC has embraced neoliberalism.

What is missing currently in many South African deliberations around poverty, inequality and health is the acceptance of the notion of a community where health services and public health are based on the values of the citizenry and, importantly, where people are encouraged to see themselves as citizens. And this voice of the citizenry needs to be heard – rather than, as currently, simply the various voices of racial and ethnic groups who promote the interests of their constituents.

This theme is picked up by Dreze and Sen (1989) in their book on hunger. They argue that avoiding hunger requires analysis not just of food intake but also of 'the person's access to health care, medical facilities, elementary education, drinking water, and sanitary facilities'. While again it would be possible to see these purely in resource terms or to 'commodify' them, the whole argument comes back to the need to have or to create the social institutions to allow these other aspects to be present, and indeed to allow such a philosophy to underpin public policy.

What is potentially problematical with respect to this view of the possible road to avoiding the neoliberal excesses of the market forces of globalisation is that South Africa has strong financial institutions and weak social institutions, many of which are a throwback to apartheid times. This issue currently gets little attention in the debate on health and health care in South Africa. The links between market economics, globalisation, increased poverty and worsening distribution of income are becoming acknowledged; the institutional weaknesses are not. What is needed in the fight against the contagion of neoliberalism through globalisation is the building of solid democratic institutions where strong unions are not only present but are accepted as key players in pacts with government and industry in deciding how the resources of a country are to be used.

One example of the failure of institutions in South Africa to protect society at large is found in the mining sector. Weston (2011) shares the disquiet of Grobler (2009), who points out that 'the Minister for Education's husband has a mining company; the Minister for Transport's wife has a mining company; the Minister for Water Affairs, who used to be the Minister of Minerals and Energy's husband, has a mining company. The Ex-Director-General of Trade and Industry and four of South Africa's provinces' previous premiers own or are BEE [Black Economic Empowerment] partners in mining companies. The list goes on and on' (Grobler 2009). Since the national election held in May 2009, the former Minister for Minerals and Energy, Buyelwa Sonjica, has been made Minister for the Environment – in other words, she will be the minister considering appeals made against the licences issued by what was formely her fief, the Department of Minerals and Energy. Environmentalists saw this as a 'sign that BEE coal-mining interests now trump environmental concerns' (Grobler 2009).

Weston, whose key concern is global warming and the mining industry, concludes:

> That such high ranking and powerful public officials benefit from the BEE programme brings into question the integrity not only of the

programme but of the overall governance of mining in South Africa. This is a major concern. The fossil fuel sector has a powerful lobbying voice at both the international level and, in the case of South Africa, at the national level where corruption and political influence merge. This is but one vignette in the case for why the elite national and global institutions will not ever tackle global warming. (Weston 2011)

To address such issues, or even to believe that they might be addressed, might seem all too difficult, but Bundorf and Fuchs give some hope. They are writing of the prospects for reform of the US health-care system:

> The same American public that voted for conservative, business-oriented governments in the 1920s embraced sweeping major shifts in economic and social policy in the 1930s. The civil rights legislation in the 1960s provides another example of major social change. We suspect, however, that the types of changes that are necessary to create strong support for a system of national health insurance are likely to be caused by significant external events. For example, a public health crisis may generate greater support for government intervention in health-care markets, even among people with unfavorable attitudes toward government intervention more generally. We think that national health insurance will come to the United States some day, but probably only in the wake of major political, economic, or social trauma, or in response to a public health crisis, continued erosion of employment-based insurance, or financial melt-down of Medicare. (2008: 24)

Some parallels with the UK

Parallels between the UK coming out of the Second World War (see Chapter 6) and post-apartheid South Africa are instructive. In both instances, the times were ripe for change not only in health care but in society in general. In the UK, the Second World War had resulted in both clearer class lines emerging and, perhaps more importantly, a louder and more cohesive working-class voice. The Labour Party Manifesto in 1945 (Labour Party 1945) reminded voters of the aftermath of the First World War: 'The people made tremendous efforts to win the last war ... but when they had won it they lacked a lively interest in the social and economic problems of peace.... The people lost that peace ... including the social and economic policy which followed the fighting.' The manifesto went on to recall how 'the hard faced men and their political friends kept control of the Government ... they controlled the banks, the mines, the big industries, largely the press and the cinema. The economic times of the 1920s and 1930s were the sure and certain result of the concentration of too much economic power in the hands of too few men.' It argued that things in 1945 had not changed and asked: 'Does freedom for the profiteer mean freedom for the ordinary man and woman?'

There is general agreement that the election of 1945 was a major turning point in British history. Social solidarity had been sufficiently strong to have a positive impact on non-combatant mortality during the war years. Amartya Sen puts this down to what he calls 'the extent of social sharing and the sharp increases in public support for social services (including nutritional support and health care) that went with this' (2001: 343).

The parallels with South Africa today are there on the negative side; the social solidarity has not yet been built.

Conclusion

The current situation in South Africa arises from the existing power structure; it is not about any rational economic analysis of priority setting. We can carry out standard health economics analyses from here to eternity and the results of these studies on their own will not shift this. These studies are needed to point the way, so to speak, but in a political economy context they are not enough. I reiterate: there needs to be a change in the power structure within the health-care system and with respect to it. That change – at least the latter change – I suggest cannot and will not occur without a change in the social and economic structure of South African society. As Lucy Gilson and I have written previously: 'With unemployment running at over 25 per cent, the economy is operating at an equilibrium that makes no economic sense. Investment is necessary but more important is to build more labour-intensive industries. The return on capital is too high and that to labour too low, thereby adding to inequality and poverty' (Mooney and Gilson 2009). That underlying imbalance is the direct result of neoliberal policies being pursued.

It would be a mistake if too many hopes were to be placed on National Health Insurance. That is no doubt important but the statistics on poverty and inequality and the gap between the beauty of the South African constitution and the ugliness of what the ANC government has become, and what it is delivering or failing to deliver to its people, question the nature of the social fabric of the South African society. The health problems are enormous. Of course they can be ameliorated through better care and especially more equitable care, but the fundamental pointers remain the two key social determinants of health or ill-health: poverty and inequality. Under neoliberalism they have got worse since the apartheid years.

8 / Australia and victim blaming

The Preventative Health Taskforce in Australia has argued for higher taxes on fast foods, cigarettes and alcohol in an attempt to get consumers to change their patterns of consumption to healthier ways. These were essentially victim-blaming policies dealing primarily with the demand side of the market with little attempt (beyond some minor suggestions such as restrictions on advertising) to change the behaviour of the perpetrators – the industries involved. This chapter charts how this happened on the policy front in tackling obesity and proposes ways in which policy could be used to influence the supply side of the obesity-inducing market.

The Preventative Health Taskforce

As is the case in many countries, Australia faces very real problems of public health around fast foods, smoking and alcohol. To address these issues, in 2008 the government set up the Preventative Health Taskforce, which was charged with making recommendations on how best to address these problems.

Encouragingly, the report quotes from a submission as follows: 'In a political economy that measures progress in terms of growth and consumption, there are many underlying environmental, social and political determinants of obesity' (Preventative Health Taskforce 2009a.: 90) Unfortunately the report does not follow through on this as might have been hoped, and does not advocate changing the political economy despite what seems on the face of it to be an identification of the political economy – of neoliberalism – as a major causal factor. It does however add: 'In this context the introduction of policy and regulatory interventions is essential to make real impacts on the prevention of obesity' (*ibid.*: 90).

When it continues – 'Changes are needed in our environments, transport systems, food supply, workplaces, schools, local communities and health-care systems to make the healthy choices the easy choices, and to empower and motivate individuals and families to lead healthier lives' – the need to change the political economy is missing from the list.

In the technical report on obesity (which was an input to the final report), in terms of addressing these political economy issues, what emerges is disappointing: 'Reshape the food supply towards lower-risk products and encourage physical activity.' This was to be done by reviewing taxation on healthy and unhealthy goods and activities, regulating the fat content in foods and subsidising fresh food in remote areas. The technical report also argued for protecting children from 'inappropriate marketing of unhealthy goods and beverages' (Preventative Health Taskforce 2009b).

I am not suggesting that these are unimportant issues. nor that addressing them will do nothing. Once again, however, they are dealing only with the symptoms rather than the underlying structural issues clearly identified in the main report – that Australia is 'a political economy that measures progress in terms of growth and consumption.'

Thus the main basis for action was to propose raising taxes and increasing prices to reduce demand and limit consumption of unhealthy commodities and unhealthy behaviours, while encouraging consumption of healthy goods and behaviours through lowered taxes.

I had thought that the Taskforce might have been restricted by its terms of reference and felt unable to delve deeper into the political economy of neoliberalism in Australia. Yet it was asked to 'address all relevant arms of policy and all available points of leverage, in both the health and non-health sectors, in formulating its recommendations' (Preventative Health Taskforce 2009a). That would, according to my reading, have allowed the committee the freedom to get into political economy issues. That they did not leads to the conclusion they chose explicitly not to go down that road.

Thus in practice the economic imperatives of the industries involved was not seen, as far as the recommendations were concerned, as a suitable entry point for interventions. The Taskforce did not recommend structural changes that might influence more fundamentally the supply side of the equation. That issue is a key consideration in this chapter.

The corporatisation of government?

The first thing that needs to be accepted about these industries is that they are there to make profits. They are not about health *per se* and in so far as they might indulge in some efforts to appear to be 'selling health', this can only be to the extent that this is perceived by the companies to increase their profits. This is because according to law the management of such companies must in all they do seek to maximise the returns to their shareholders. Anything else such as image building is not an end in itself; it is a process undertaken to increase profits. It has to be. As lawyer David Ritter (2011) notes: 'By law, companies must maximise returns to shareholders, a legal obligation that is brutally reinforced by the economic reality of the ultra-competitive globalised marketplace.'

It is noteworthy that in arguing this and in his cynicism about what is euphemistically called 'social responsibility', Ritter quotes none other than Milton Friedman, the guru of neoliberalism:

> '[I]n practice the doctrine of social responsibility is frequently a cloak for actions that are justified on other grounds rather than a reason for those actions.... To illustrate, it may well be in the long run interest of a corporation that is a major employer in a small community to devote resources to providing amenities to that community or to improving its government.

He gives various examples but then adds: 'In each of these – and many similar – cases, there is a strong temptation to rationalise these actions as an exercise of "social responsibility".... [T]his is one way for a corporation to generate goodwill as a by-product of expenditures that are entirely justified in its own self-interest.'

This is not to deny that it is better for companies to maximise their own interests by doing good rather than doing evil. I just want to be clear that the motivation of management has to be seen in terms of doing good for their company. The question that then arises is whether, when a government is seeking advice on health issues in food policy, it is appropriate to have food industry representatives involved. Given the necessity for companies to seek to work only in the interests of the companies' shareholders, the answer would seem to be no. In any conflict that might arise (and that is inevitable) between the interests of the company and the public interest, the former is more likely to win.

Yet this happens. In the UK, for example, the government has argued that issues such as obesity are everyone's business and consequently businesses involved in food production such as McDonald's and Pepsi should have a hand in devising government food policy.

Thus:

> Fast food companies including McDonald's and Kentucky Fried Chicken have been invited by the Department of Health to help write government policy on obesity, alcohol and diet-related disease.... Processed food and drink manufacturers including PepsiCo, Kellogg's, Unilever, Mars and Diageo are also among the businesses that have been asked to contribute to five 'responsibility deal' networks set up by Health Secretary Andrew Lansley. (*Daily Mail* 2010)

It is not surprising that those concerned about the public's health have been critical. For example Professor Anna Gilmore, a public health expert from Bath University, has said 'there is a fundamental conflict of interest that has been ignored' (Hughes 2011). She goes on: 'These large corporations, whether they sell tobacco, food or alcohol, are legally obliged to maximise shareholder returns. They therefore have to oppose any policies that could reduce sales and profitability – in other words, the most effective policies.'

In Australia a somewhat similar situation arose with the Preventative Health Taskforce membership regarding industry being invited to participate in policy making, although perhaps the conflict of interest was not as extreme as in the UK example quoted above. Appointed to that taskforce was Ms Kate Carnell who, after her appointment, joined the Australian Food and Grocery Council as chief executive. This is the industry lobby group, as their website claims: 'We are the leading national organisation representing Australia's packaged food, drink and grocery products manufacturers. Our role is to help shape a business environment that encourages the food and grocery products industry to grow and remain profitable' (see www.afgc.org.au/whoweare.html). It was a controversial appointment.

It was also very firmly and explicitly supported by Nicola Roxon, the Australian Health Minister, who included the following in a speech to the Australian Food and Grocery Council Dinner on 28 October 2009:

> I must also take this opportunity to acknowledge the role that Kate Carnell has played as a member of the Taskforce, and thank her and all Taskforce members for their hard work. In this room, you will know there was some criticism about Kate remaining on the Taskforce when she took this new role. But I have a high regard for Kate's ability, and *I saw no reason for people to fear industry engagement – quite the opposite.* (Roxon 2009; italics added).

It is also the case that Ms Carnell on behalf of her organisation and in defence of the situation in which she found herself indicated that 'the industry has introduced front-of-pack labels – listing the recommended daily intake (RDI) of nutrients the product represents – to help consumers make informed choices'. But the eminent nutritionist Rosemary Stanton branded this RDI system 'a total and complete nonsense' (Stark 2009).

What is also remarkable in Australia and New Zealand is that of the 12 members of the board of the Food Standards Australia and New Zealand, no fewer than five hold or have held senior positions in the food industry. This is the government body which regulates the content and labelling of food in these two countries.

Thus these industries, which very clearly are a major part of the problem of obesity, are directly involved in setting government policy on food. This is despite the fact that the people involved from these companies have a clear legal obligation to do the best they can for their shareholders. In the UK there has been some vociferous opposition from the public health lobby against this involvement by industry. In Australia, while the criticism has been more muted, the health minister has gone out of her way to praise the food industry representative on the Preventative Health

Taskforce. The links between corporations and government are very clear, explicit and welcomed by government – even when, in the case of the food industry, the health of the public is at stake.

So what might be done?

There is a need ideally for a new political economy. That is spelt out in some detail later, in Chapter 12. That will not happen soon. What is clear is that the majority of the public recognise obesity is a problem, and this is a good start if they are to become more involved in setting policy to do something about it. Thus, in the short run, we can attempt to tap into what the critically informed community wants.

Beyond that, and without being too radical, what I have proposed with my colleague Todd Harper is to tax the advertising and marketing budgets of fast food producers by a large amount, perhaps 100 per cent (Harper and Mooney 2010). That tax would vary depending on how harmful the products were to health. Thus the higher the harm, the higher the tax. This is addressing the supply side issue.

If the companies did not change their behaviour, this would mean that consumers would face higher prices, as the companies might be assumed to pass on most if not all of the tax in higher prices. Alternatively the companies would be faced with an incentive to reduce their tax. They could reduce their advertising budget or they could lower the harm content of their product, or most profitably tackle both aspects. As for the consumers, they would either face less advertising and, assuming the company had previously been acting rationally in seeking profit maximisation, reduce their consumption; or they would be consuming less harmful fare.

The idea was taken up by the Greens Party (a strong but minority party in Australia), but not by the major parties. What is striking is that there was so little attempt to address the most fundamental issue in this sort of economy – all that can be done on the supply side is to try to restrict the advertising of companies and use price signals on the demand side to limit consumption. That may 'work', but that is not the point I want to make.

But before I turn to that, we should note that the consumption of fast foods is now very much dominated by the poor. The impact of raising prices risks creating a situation where the poor are pushed further into poverty. It is also a policy which is very much about blaming the victim, and is supported mainly by middle-class people, many of whom no doubt bemoan the fact that these people do not behave like them.

Such victim blaming cannot be good for self-esteem or in turn for health. Indeed it is worth noting that in a citizens' jury that I facilitated (ACT Health Council 2010) there was a quite lengthy debate about what recommendations to make regarding the growing problem of obesity in Australia. (Citizens' juries are a form of deliberative democracy which involves bringing together randomly selected citizens, giving them good information, and then asking them to deliberate as citizens representing their community on an issue or issues. They then make recommendations about what they as representatives of their community want. More detail on citizens' juries is provided in Chapter 13.) Initially the discussion centred on the question of raising prices through higher taxes on fast foods, which essentially echoed what the Preventative Health Taskforce had come up with. But then one young woman who had worked in the slimming industry argued that most of the clients she had seen had some emotional problems which had resulted in their bad eating habits: they were stressed because of marital problems, or their kids were playing up, or they were being bullied at work. What was needed, she argued, was to address these problems. The obesity was a symptom of a deeper malaise.

What that jury recommended on this front was 'strongly supporting illness prevention/health promotion as an area for increased funding' (ACT Health Council 2010). They highlighted the importance of understanding why people adopt unhealthy behaviours so that prevention measures are more helpful, pointing out that preventative measures must avoid blaming or penalising the victim.

> Jurors referred to obesity as an example and stressed that there are often underlying problems that lead to unhealthy behaviours, which will not be addressed by merely advising people to eat less. Simply telling people that junk food was bad for them was unlikely to be effective and could lead to resentment.

Jurors also did not want extra taxes to be imposed on consumers – rather they wanted disincentives to be aimed at manufacturers and vendors. (ACT Health Council 2010)

Out of the mouths of 'ordinary' (but critically informed) citizens ...!

Conclusion

This chapter has highlighted two key issues. First it has drawn attention to the tendency in policy on health promotion and health prevention to blame the victim, while not addressing the problems created by industry in a neoliberal economy. Second, it has shown how governments are captured by the perpetrators of harmful (in this instance, obesity-inducing) industries, something that is often the case in public health and in most areas of concern to everyone. As Nicola Roxon, the Australian Health Minister put it, she 'saw no reason for people to fear industry engagement – quite the opposite'.

'Quite the opposite'? Really?

9 / **Local community versus corporation**

This chapter tells the story of the small town of Yarloop and its fight with its neighbour, the alumina corporation Alcoa and its Wagerup refinery. It tells of how this unequal battle was supported on only one side – the corporation's – by government. Despite the fact that there was good evidence of adverse health effects from pollution, the community lost. The case study shows how governments – and also universities – can be 'captured' by corporations.

Health policy and the corporatisation of government

This chapter draws on the book by Martin Brueckner and Dyann Ross (2010). It is a most useful account of aspects of this saga. One of the themes running through their book is the extent to which in health policy (and indeed policy in other sectors as well) there has been what is perhaps best described as 'a corporatisation of government'. It is an important issue and one that has changed markedly since the advent of neoliberalism in the late 1970s. The market has taken over the state and, as Harvey (2005) remarks, while it is often stated that neoliberalism is about the withering away of the state and the rise of small government, these are poor descriptors of the reality of what has happened to the state. If we go back in time to the view of Keynes, it is clear that he saw a major role for the state (see Spartacus Educational nd). Significantly, it was the role of a benevolent state which sought to act in the interests of the people it represented – the public. He did not foresee the way in which the state would be captured by corporations. As will become clear it is not just government which is thus captured; other social institutions, such as universities,

94

can suffer the same fate. Others still, such as the churches, many NGOs, health services, schools, sports and the media are, even if not captured, nonetheless heavily influenced by and often heavily financially supported by corporations.

Today, all too often, it is 'big business' which dictates or heavily influences what governments do. Many corporations are international, hence 'TNCs' – transnational corporations – control resources which are massive, even in terms of substantial countries' national incomes. For example:

> With over 53 per cent of the world's largest economies today being transnational corporations (TNCs) their impact and responsibilities are global and it is crucial that they be held accountable for the numerous violations which are being perpetrated on a daily basis in the name of maximising production and profits. In 2006 total sales of the top 200 transnational corporations were bigger than the combined GDP of 187 countries, more than 30 per cent of world GDP, while they employ less than a third of the world population. (Foundation of Gaia, no date)

It is useful to put these issues into perspective in ways that connect with the lives of sometimes quite small local communities, as the global dimensions can at times get overwhelming. The story of Yarloop, a small community in Western Australia, provides that perspective.

Yarloop, Alcoa and the corporatisation of the West Australian government

Yarloop is a small town of 600 people to the south of Perth, the state capital of Western Australia. In 1984 the US-based company Alcoa began operating its alumina refinery just 2 kilometres from Yarloop. In Western Australia it has 4,000 employees.

As Brueckner and Ross report, 'Since the mid-1990s, residents and Alcoa workers have reported symptoms such as frequent blood noses, headaches and nausea.' They add: 'No causal link has been formally established between the refinery's emissions and people's health' (2010: 21). Then in 2006 'the state government approved a major expansion at the Wagerup refinery – despite community concerns and reservations voiced by the WA Health Department as well as independent medical experts' (*ibid.*: 23).

It is important to recognise that Western Australia is a big mining state and that much of the economic prosperity not only of the state but the country comes from the likes of Alcoa. When it was originally established 'the [earlier] Court government was reported to have been "exploring every possible avenue to bring the ... project to fruition" calling its eventual establishment "a great moment for WA and the nation"' (*ibid*.: 41). When concerns emerged about possible health effects from the refinery, 'the state government formed the Wagerup Medical Practitioners' Forum to discuss and investigate health problems in Alcoa workers and community members' (*ibid*.: 47).

The situation and the political economy underlying what happened at Yarloop is summed up in this excerpt from Brueckner and Ross:

> The development maxim adhered to by successive state governments in Western Australia has placed at risk the sustainability of a small community, which due to no fault of its own came too close to the engines of the state economy. The government's economic credo, coupled with the relative electoral insignificance of the Yarloop area, effectively overrode local concerns about the refinery. Yet the approach by government was consistent with the neoliberal, economic rationalist stance which accepts and advocates the primacy of the markets and believes in small government and big business. Indeed, the state government, itself a beneficiary of economic growth, appears as an almost invisible stakeholder in the conflict. Ministerial decisions and departmental responses to refinery-related matters only served to fuel local perceptions of collusion which were echoed by political insiders. (*Ibid*.: 251)

In the context of the Wagerup site and its expansion, the independent members of the Wagerup Medical Practitioners' Forum (2005) made a submission to the Environmental Protection Authority regarding the health effects of the proposed expansion. The WMPF are a group of distinguished medical doctors who are 'independent from industry and government'.

They made a number of points in their submission. These included:

> The history of workers at the existing refinery, in our professional opinion, shows that some workers have suffered acute and chronic adverse health consequences as the result of working at the refinery....

The available evidence indicates that some of the neighbouring community members, including the people in the township of Yarloop, in our professional opinion, have suffered acute and chronic adverse health consequences as a result of the close proximity of the existing refinery....

Alcoa was initially slow to respond to these health problems, and, while Alcoa's responsiveness has improved, there has been insufficient duration or consistency of an improved performance on this issue to give us confidence that Alcoa has accepted ownership of the problems.

They cite a number of reasons for this view and conclude that 'the initiative to address new illness among workers and the community has been taken by workers and the community, rather than by Alcoa.'

Andrew Harper, a member of the Medical Practitioners' Forum, expressed concern about the way in which some of the medical advice was sought by Alcoa, especially around the question of what is known as 'multiple chemical sensitivity': 'The doctors who were brought over [from the east of Australia] by Alcoa were very critical of the treating doctors involved ... but I do not think they helped the situation at all, I think that was very much a negative and a hostile way of behaving.'

As it happens, one of these doctors, Julian Lee, suggested that this condition was not a disease. He went further. To say it was, he argued, was 'doing [those so diagnosed] a great disservice, and in fact may well interfere with their health, their welfare, their economic independence, a whole range of criteria that can impact upon people when you're given a misdiagnosis' (Background Briefing ABC 2002).

Dr Chrissy Sharp, who was then a member of the state parliament, chaired a three-year-long Western Australian Legislative Council Inquiry into the Alcoa Refinery at Wagerup. However before her committee reported, the state government allowed Alcoa to proceed with its application for expansion. Interviewed by ABC *Four Corners* (2005), she said she was was 'bitterly disappointed.'

Alcoa has a very close relationship with the state government. Alcoa is one of the biggest players in the West Australian economy ... has enormous influence ... and has done for a long time. The State Agreement Acts that it operates under have enormous advantages to the company. It doesn't pay all sorts of rates and taxes that would be expected. For example its revenue, its royalty base is very low indeed ... so they've got a good deal here and that is why the alumina industry has come to focus on the South West ... we offer stability ... we offer state governments that will bend over backwards to allow these kinds of big enterprises to be established and to enjoy stability.

Sharp argued that there was a need for an independent research study of the emissions from Wagerup which, astonishingly given the background to this issue, had not taken place (and at the time of writing still has not taken place). She went on to reveal that such a research programme 'has been rejected by Alcoa on the grounds of cost'. She argued that that 'seems extraordinary' for such a rich company. 'You would have thought they could find the million dollars to do this research programme.' She also expressed disappointment that the state government had taken the view that the research programme was unnecessary. She argued that government had shown total contempt in allowing the expansion when they had not heard from her committee, whose report was due shortly thereafter.

We were the parliament (committee) investigating something independent of the executive government, and there was government turning around and saying, we're not really interested in your views, we'll make sure that they become irrelevant, and that we're going to collaborate with an industry in order that they achieve their ambitions, rather than give proper respect to good parliamentary work.

University capture

The reach of conglomerates like Alcoa can be vast. Within this particular tale, I also want to highlight at a more personal level the way in which Alcoa was able to influence the university in which I was employed in Western Australia. It may be more accurate to suggest that it was the university management's perception of what Alcoa might do that was the influence here. That may be a rather fine distinction; what matters is that the influence is a reality – whether direct and explicit, or subtle and perceived.

With respect to my own involvement, relevant here is a report from the Australia Institute (Hamilton and Downie 2007) which looked at university capture by the fossil fuel industry in Western Australia. This industry is massive in the state and makes a major contribution to the Australian GNP. It has a lot of power. When for example in 2009 the Labour government under then Prime Minister Kevin Rudd tried to introduce a mining tax on excess profits, the industry mounted a multi-million-dollar campaign against the tax and forced the government first to withdraw it, second to redraw it, and third to water it down to a level acceptable to the industry. Many argue that it was the attack by the mining industry on his attempt to introduce this tax that was a major factor in Kevin Rudd being forced out and replaced by Julia Gillard as prime minister. The power over the Australian government (and others – see for example Patrick Bond 2005 on the power of the South African fossil industry over governments there) is very great.

With respect to 'university capture', what Hamilton and Downie (2007) showed is that in Australia, and particularly in the resource-rich state of Western Australia, a number of universities have been captured by the fossil fuel industries. They examined four. The links between these universities and the fossil fuel industries are deep and flow through many conduits.

Regarding the university that I worked at in Western Australia, Curtin University, the authors state that Woodside [a major oil and gas company in the state] is

> prominent at Curtin University. Curtin is home to the Woodside Hydrocarbon Research Facility and the Chair of Hydrocarbon Research, both funded by the company. It is also the location for the Western Australian Energy Research Alliance, a joint venture in part funded by Woodside and Chevron Texaco, and the Centre of Excellence in Cleaner Production supported by Wesfarmers. The Chancellor of the university is on the boards of a major oil and gas company. There is also an Alcoa Research Centre for Stronger Communities – funded by Alcoa, the major alumina transnational corporation.

This sort of university capture is of course not unique to Australia. The New Economics Foundation argued in 2003 that many of Britain's top universities 'could be brought into disrepute' by 'walking hand-in-hand' with fossil fuel companies (quoted in Hamilton and Downie 2007).

What is also worrying is that in carrying out their research on university capture Hamilton and Downie struggled to get academics to speak up. I did, but this was late in my career and, had it been earlier, and had I been more junior at the time, I am not sure I would have been as willing to speak up and be quoted.

With respect to Curtin University and Alcoa, I met some of the people of Yarloop when I was involved in a health service conference (not on their plight), discovered some of the health problems they faced, and so began to take an interest in the issue. I then discovered that Alcoa had a centre researching into community development at my university. That centre was mentioned in *The West Australian*, the local state newspaper, by their leading journalist Paul Murray, who drew attention to the health problems of the people of Yarloop and to the fact that it was of note that the company against which the local people were complaining was also funding this 'stronger communities' centre at Curtin.

Murray was also the presenter on a local radio programme and in that capacity invited me to be interviewed about the links between Alcoa and Curtin. I accepted. Part of what I said (the rest was in similar vein) was as follows:

> If it is the case that a community or its representatives want to get some advice or get some evaluation done ... or something or other, it's very important that they know that they can go to an independent source for that, such as a university. My worry, and the worry of a lot of academics at the present time, is that by getting into bed with the corporates, that independence may be, in a sense, challenged. And indeed, there may be a perception that it should be challenged.

Later on that day, I was given a talking-to by senior management at my university and very clearly told that there was unhappiness at my 'disloyalty' to the university in talking to this journalist. I took this to be more about concerns about a possible withdrawal of funds by Alcoa and others who might have seen that academics at Curtin were prepared to speak out about possible adverse effects on the community of companies who put funding into research at Curtin University.

Hamilton and Downie reported:

> the administration at Curtin University expressed its displeasure when a professor at the university spoke publicly about Alcoa's funding of

the Alcoa Research Centre for Stronger Communities at the University, at the same time as the company was being criticised in the media over pollution from one of its plants damaging the health of a local community. (2007: vi)

I am not suggesting that Curtin is the only university behaving in this way. It has to be the case, however, that many academics in such a climate, especially those earlier in their careers than I was, would be wary of speaking out. It is difficult to imagine that a member of the Alcoa Centre for Stronger Communities would be openly critical of Alcoa's seemingly unsympathetic position regarding the complaints from Yarloop residents, as documented above. They might, but the probability would surely be greater if the money for that centre came from government.

In this particular situation that possibility was never going to occur anyway, as I only discovered later in reading *Under Corporate Skies*. As Brueckner and Ross reveal, 'we were told that the new Centre was not going to be addressing the specifics of the Wagerup issue'.

Hamilton and Downie write: 'One of the roles of university lecturers and researchers ... is to use their expertise to assess and comment on the practices of industry.... However if these academics or their universities are employed by or have financial association with ... companies [in these industries] then they may well feel constrained or gagged'. The authors claim, I believe justifiably, that the evidence they present 'indicates that there are grounds for concern as commercial interests are intertwined in universities'.

Conclusion

There are many issues that are troubling in this case study and they all revolve around the impact of corporate power on people's lives but also on the corporatisation of government. I chose to focus on the latter in the chapter, although other issues are perhaps just as worrying.

The story of Yarloop is very much a David and Goliath story, with Goliath having two heads – the corporation Alcoa and the Western Australian state government. In this state the resources industry is important economically. As a result it has become just as important politically. It undermines democracy at many levels from the state itself to small communities like Yarloop. It threatens health and well-being, and the integrity of our universities and our academics. It ought not to be so, but under neoliberalism it is.

Many of the people of Yarloop fight on; others have given up; and yet others have moved out. There will now never be an adequate inquiry to establish the full facts. Such an inquiry would only be in the interests of the people of Yarloop.

10 / The pharmaceutical industry

In Chapter 7 I reported on the fight between the South African government and the big pharmaceutical companies. At a broader level this is an issue that goes on constantly, with Big Pharma by and large neglecting the diseases of the poor. Under the terms of capitalism and neoliberalism this is hardly surprising. Trying to sell drugs to the poor is hard simply because they are poor. Profit maximisation will not happen if companies adopt such a sales campaign. It might be good for image building and hence for profits if a company indulges in some seemingly charitable work to aid the poor, but given the legal framework under which they operate they simply cannot get into good works for charitable purposes.

This situation is reflected in figures from Barnard (2002: 163–4) regarding drug sales in Africa. He writes:

> Despite the fact that Africa contains approximately 13 per cent of the world's total population, at the time of this lawsuit African drug sales by multinational pharmaceutical corporations represented only 1 per cent of worldwide sales. This reflects what has been termed the 'global drug gap', in which weak market incentives and weak to nonexistent local industrial capacity combine to create ever widening disparities between rich and poor nations in the availability and development of drugs. Investments for research and development in the pharmaceutical industry follow market incentives closely. An assessment of 1,233 new drugs coming to market between 1975 and 1997, for example, identified only 13 products approved specifically for tropical diseases. (Reich 2000)

What to do?

Strictly the problem is not the drug companies; it is the economic imperatives of capitalism which drive companies to behave in this way. There is little point in blaming the industry when they are simply playing by the rules. We need to change the rules. I will say more of this in the concluding chapter but, as Barnard argues, 'substantial improvements in population health in the developing world will depend on developing shared goals among the rich and poor nations, social and economic policies to improve living and working conditions – especially to promote education, equality, and empowerment of women – sustainable economic development, and ongoing research into the root causes of poor population health and their pathways of action'.

No one would seriously dispute that fine sentiment, but unfortunately Barnard does not tell us how to get there. That is the challenge that I have tried to pick up. That notion of shared goals based on equality and the promotion of social improvement is the basis of communitarian claims as laid out later in Chapter 12. I return to the practical implications of these goals in the Conclusion.

The lengths to which the pharmaceutical industry will go to pursue profits is nonetheless quite extraordinary at times. It is also important to note that often their behaviour requires others to respond positively or even just naïvely to their overtures. It happens so often. But every now and then Big Pharma manages to find yet more offensive ways of trying to corrupt research, clinicians and the WHO.

They do so against a background of truly massive profits. As Marcia Angell, a former editor of the prestigious *New England Journal of Medicine*, writes, for 2002 the combined profits of the ten drug companies in the US on the 'Fortune 500' – the top US companies – 'were more than the profits of all the other 490 businesses put together ... When I say this is a profitable industry, I mean really profitable. It is difficult to conceive of how awash in money Big Pharma is.' She also notes that 'drug industry expenditures for research and development, while large, were consistently far less than profits' and that what goes into 'marketing and administration' is 'two and a half times the expenditures for R & D' (Angell 2004: 11–12).

Reacting to Big Pharma

Some in health services – doctors and others – remain willing to take the Big Pharma shilling without any recognition of the conflicts of interests involved. Here are a couple of examples from my own experience. Nearly 20 years ago, a leading Australian clinician was keen to do a study with me which would have involved bringing a colleague out from the UK. He said he'd get the money for the airfare from a drug company. I indicated that if there was any drug company money involved then I would not be. He was amazed at this response and said: 'I can't remember when I last paid for an airfare.'

More recently I suggested to a very senior university administrator that the university should not accept drug company money when evaluating drugs, since there was good evidence that such funding resulted in bias in favour of the company's drug. 'Studies sponsored by pharmaceutical companies were more likely to have outcomes favouring the sponsor than were studies with other sponsors' (Lexchin *et al.* 2003). The university administrator's response? 'But if we say no, Gavin, the company will just go down the road to another university!'

More seriously, a colleague published an article in a prestigious peer-reviewed medical journal which looked at the relative cost-effectiveness of various options for a particular condition. One of these was a medicine intervention. He found that the medicine intervention did not do well compared to the others and reported this finding in his article. Shortly thereafter, he was contacted by the head of the government agency which used such publications to guide it in its policy making regarding recommendations for the use of different pharmaceutical products. He had received advice from two leading academics regarding the product covered by my colleague's study. They both sought to 'rubbish' the study and expressed surprise that the prestigious journal should have agreed to publish the article. My colleague would never have known this but for the fact that he knew the head of the agency involved. I know the article and my assessment is that it contains a thorough, rigorous analysis, but more importantly at least two reviewers for that journal agreed with that assessment.

I do not of course know quite why such events occurred but I harbour my suspicions. Other such events make me think that there is a pattern here. At least some academic researchers are capable of being influenced when they act as consultants to particular organisations. There has to be a better way for our pharmaceutical industries to do business. My point is that that better way does not exist under a neoliberal regime. There is a need for a new system of incentives. We need a new political economy.

There are such stories on a much bigger scale. One is the recent case of WHO and the swine flu pandemic. Ramesh (2010) reported: 'An investigation by the *British Medical Journal* and the Bureau of Investigative Journalism ... shows that WHO guidance [on stock-piling drugs in the event of a flu pandemic] issued in 2004 was authored by three scientists who had previously received payment for other work from Roche ... and GlaxoSmithKline (GSK)' – the companies that make the drugs which were to be stockpiled. The guidance led to drug companies making billions of dollars from the stockpiling.

Another related aspect of this is that many doctors are involved in research, for example in testing out new drugs. The results of this research are then written up in articles in medical journals and in turn often used to influence health-care policy. Clearly if the industry were able to influence the writing of these articles, then that might well increase their sales, which would hence be in the interests of their shareholders.

Do they? They do, and this can happen in various ways. The most infamous examples are the ghost writing of articles by what are known as 'medical communication agencies'. These agencies are employed by the pharmaceutical industry to draft articles which are then passed on to doctors to put their names to for publication in scientific journals. While this practice may not be known to the general public, within health policy circles it has been known about for years.

And it still goes on. An article in the British newspaper *The Guardian* (Ross 2011) quotes a medical writer who has worked for 'medical communication agencies' (read firms of ghost writers). He tells of how an article he wrote about a new cancer treatment will appear in print later this year 'with an oncologist considered a "key opinion leader" listed as the author in his stead'. He is quoted as saying: 'You'd do the same thing if you were selling cornflakes. It's no different'.

What is also concerning is that most of this research in 'clinical trials' is paid for not by the taxpayer but by the industry! One might be cynical and think that such industry funding might bias the results in favour of the industry's products. Unfortunately such cynicism is justified. A number of studies have shown that industry-funded research is more likely to show that a pharmaceutical product is effective in its treatment. The 'best' example is reported by Gupta and Cohen (2010):

> Researchers from the United States and Canada looked at 546 drug trials ... 346 of them, or 63 per cent, were funded by the drug industry. The remaining 200 were paid for by government or non-profit organizations. Study authors found that more than 85 per cent of the industry-funded trials in their sample posted favorable outcomes and were 4 times more likely to report findings that favored their drug.

Again, trying to stop this sort of behaviour even if we see it as abhorrent is difficult in a neoliberal world. As Angell remarks, 'What is the mission of an academic medical center? Surely it's not to serve the drug companies. But increasingly that's how the academic medical centers see themselves' (quoted in Reynolds 2001: 1592).

Can this sort of corruption be stopped? Well there seems not much point in trying to stop individual clinical researchers and individual universities accepting payment and kickbacks from the drug companies. It's been tried. It does not work. Policing it is impossible and the climate and culture of clinical research would need a revolution.

The place to tackle this is in the incentive structures that the industry faces in this neoliberal world. State ownership of companies is one option. Those who worry that investment in new drugs would dry up need to note that currently only 14 per cent of the industry's budgets goes on developing drugs (Angell 2004). Another attractive option is one that economist Joseph Stiglitz (2006) has suggested. He proposes a massive multi-billion-dollar prize be set up by governments which would be awarded on the basis of drug inventions which did the most to improve health. I would suggest that rather than have governments pay for the prize, as Stiglitz proposes, that this is funded by taxing the drug companies' marketing budgets.

The way in which pharmaceutical companies can act to try to maximise their profits, but within the legal framework set by the WTO, is exemplified in their use of patents. We need to realise two things. First, the argument for having a patent law to protect companies is accepted as being important not only for the companies involved but in respect of social well-being as well. If a company invests heavily in research to produce some new product, then it needs to be assured that it will get some reasonable return on that investment – or it will probably not carry out the research. It wants to know that other companies cannot quickly come along and 'steal' its profits by producing a similar product. So patents protect companies for some years from being faced with this sort of stealing. Thus patents, when they work well, are about trying to get the optimal amount of research conducted.

Against that background the following case is worrying.

> The San people ... live in the Kalahari desert in South Africa, Botswana, Namibia and Angola. The San chew the *hoodia* ... plant on hunting expeditions because they have learned that it can help suppress their appetite. A South African research institute and a UK-based company patented the plant's key constituents and then sold the rights to develop and market the resulting drug for millions of dollars to Pfizer, a powerful pharmaceutical company. The San people were not consulted during this process. (Health Poverty Action 2011)

Only after an international campaign did the San win the rights to share in the profits made from their traditional knowledge. But the percentage they will receive is only a tiny proportion of net sales.

This is theft. It is also bizarre that anyone would want to patent something that occurs naturally. It is even more bizarre that such theft was allowed and a patent awarded. This example is again not unique. Perhaps the most 'celebrated' example is the attempt to patent the seed for basmati rice Raghavan (2000). The fact that the

WTO under the TRIPS Agreement allows these thefts to occur is an indictment of the neoliberal principles that organisation seeks to uphold.

Conclusion

Of course pharmaceutical companies are in the business of making as much profit for their shareholders as they can. That is their goal. Of course they can provide very substantial health benefits. That is not an issue.

If they have the opportunity to persuade more doctors to use more of their products, then of course the industry will try. That is fair enough: but health services, doctors, politicians and the public in general need to understand better the neoliberal objectives which the pharmaceutical companies have, and then act accordingly. A recent local case here in Western Australia opens up some of the issues we need to confront.

Pharmaceutical companies were paying for travel and accommodation for doctors to attend conferences overseas. When this arrangement was exposed, the state's director general for health responded by saying that the companies involved had in each case signed an agreement that there was no obligation on the conference attendee to do anything to benefit the company. It was also argued that such attendance at conferences was in the interests of the doctor's patients. But while the first justification is just naïve, the second statement, if true, indicates that the taxpayer should be paying for such travel. It can be important for doctors to keep up to date by attending conferences to learn about new developments in pharmaceuticals and other medical advances. But there need to be transparent limits. Most of the information on these developments quickly gets into the medical journals and doctors can readily learn from these sources. There is another problem here. If a doctor is at a conference, he or she cannot be treating patients. Doctors do need to keep up to date, but much more transparency is needed about how such travel is paid for, and what the optimal amount of conference attendance is. The Big Pharma companies are not charitable organisations. They are profit-seeking. If the industry pays for someone to go to a conference in Paris or Los Angeles or wherever, they do so because they think it is in their shareholders' interests. It is as simple as that.

The majority of health problems in this world are in very poor countries where there are very limited monies available from governments and from people to pay for drugs. So the chances currently of neoliberally run Big Pharma seeking to develop drugs for developing countries are remote – the prospect of making profits is just not there. So the R & D on malaria drugs, for example, is inevitably tiny. And the extent to which the world gets on top of malaria is ... tiny.

Here again the corporatisation of governments is all too apparent, as the following example from Wikileaks shows. To try to lower the price of drugs to their citizens, the government of Ecuador in 2009 sought to bring in compulsory licensing which 'authorises generic competition with patented, monopoly protected drugs' (Public Citizen 2011). According to international protocols, Ecuador can only do this for 'medical conditions that are priorities for public health'. Despite this,

> cables from US Embassy personnel in Ecuador to the US Department of State, released by Wikileaks, show the United States, multinational pharmaceutical companies, and three ministers within the government shared information and worked to undermine Ecuador's emerging policy ... the US mission in Quito [Ecuador's capital] explored organising wealthy countries with patent-based pharmaceutical industries against Ecuador's policy. (*Ibid.*)

Fortunately, they failed. Currently the world's poor struggle to pay for their drugs. When they succeed they often push themselves deeper into poverty. When they fail, they die.

11 / Neoliberalism and global warming

In 2009 the leading medical journal *The Lancet* published a major and much-quoted review of the impact of global warming on health (Costello *et al.* 2009). In an editorial it argued that: 'Climate change is the biggest global health threat of the twenty-first century' (*The Lancet* 2009).

Ever since temperature measurement began in the middle of the nineteenth century, temperatures have been rising. In the last thirty years, however, there has been a much faster increase. Various scientific papers in the last few years have predicted 'tipping points' in global warming. After we reach these, there will be a 'feedback' which results in global warming gathering pace, whatever we as humans then do (Lenton *et al.* 2008) – in other words, we will be able to do nothing to stop it. As Weston (2011) predicts: 'If it has not already happened, it is now almost certain that within several years we will have set in motion sufficient feedback mechanisms so that humans will be powerless to stop the Earth's change to a new climate and possibly a new geological era which will not be conducive to human life.'

Until recently climate scientists have claimed that we needed to keep global warming to a rise of less than 2°c, but key scientists (Anderson and Bows 2011; Hansen *et al.* 2008) now suggest that this represents potential global disaster, with the former contending that 'despite high-level statements to the contrary, there is now little to no chance of maintaining the global mean surface temperature at or below [a rise of] 2°c'.

This chapter argues three points. First, the fact of global warming and its impact on health urgently needs to be set in a political economy framework. Second, it is here that we shall find the source

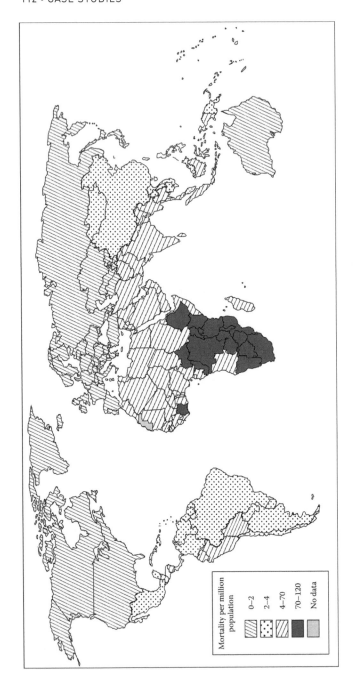

Estimated deaths attributed to climate change in the year 2000, by subregion

Data source: McMichael *et al.* (2004).

of global warming – in capitalist and neoliberal development. Third, the chapter highlights that capitalism cannot solve the problem of global warming – and indeed that we have to find new ways of organising societies and economies to maintain the planet as liveable for the future.

Global warming, health and political economy

Costello *et al.* (2009: 1963) state: 'Effects of climate change on health will affect most populations in the next decades and put the lives and well-being of billions of people at increased risk.' They add that 'the poorest countries will suffer the greatest consequences of climate change even though they contributed the least to emissions.' They show that even in the year 2000 climate change was responsible for 5.5 million disability-adjusted life years (DALYs) lost.

These findings are confirmed graphically in the map opposite.

As indicated, particularly vulnerable is sub-Saharan Africa, which even in the year 2000 was showing deaths attributable to climate change at rates of between 70 and 120 per million population, compared to between 0 and 2 per million in many Western countries. These sorts of differentials between rich and poor countries, but at higher levels, will continue into the future.

For the purposes of this chapter, however, it is what Costello *et al.* go on to say on the economic front that is critical. 'The current financial crisis raises doubts about a global model to reduce inequities based on economic growth. Contraction and convergence increase the need for new economic approaches, which place sustainability and equity at the centre of the economic debate' (2009: 1712). The doubts they express about the current economic system's failure to deal with inequities and their call for 'new economic approaches' indicate they have no faith in 'a global model ... based on economic growth' – that is, capitalism.

This is truly fascinating. Costello and his distinguished colleagues, no group of radicals, are basically calling for the abandonment of the neoliberal agenda globally. They are asking for a new political economy to save the planet. They do not specify what that might be and it would be too much to expect them to do so, but some elements are implicitly present. It would, for example, be concerned with reducing inequality and would focus less on the individual and more on social and cultural values. Sustainability would be key.

What is also of interest is that while their article has been much discussed and quoted, little attention seems to have been given to their call for 'new economic approaches'. Yet in terms of the debate around global warming, in particular around its health effects, and considerations of possible solutions, this call for a new economic system based on 'sustainability and equity' has to be one of the most important issues raised in their article.

For example, in the wake of a series of articles published in *The Lancet*, that journal presented an 'executive summary' (*The Lancet* nd) with 18 'key messages'. Not one of these, however, refers to the call for 'new economic approaches'; nor do any of them draw on the concerns expressed by Costello and his colleagues about the inability of the current economic system to address global warming. Is denialism present here too?

The past and continuing impact of neoliberalism on global warming is massive. But neoliberalism is not only a problem in being the main architect of global warming; it is a problem at the level of possible solutions. The main contender here is carbon pricing, which is a market mechanism that will almost certainly fail. Further, while that kind of mechanism is being tried, scarce time is being lost in trying to come up with solutions that might work.

How did it happen?

The source of global warming is the lust for more and more, faster and faster, economic growth. That in turn has been and continues to be driven by the growth in the use of energy and in particular of fossil fuels, the impact of which on carbon emissions is literally devastating for the planet. We are now, according to the best scientific evidence available, close to the point where we cannot stop global warming. We cannot do enough, nor quickly enough, to save the planet through renewables. We must slow or even reverse economic growth and the only way to do that is to find a non-capitalist economic model.

The unfortunate thing is that, while it is capitalism and more recently and more crucially neoliberalism that have brought about this impending disaster, there is still a common belief that market solutions are possible. We need a much more radical solution. We need to abandon capitalism. In the industrialised West we need to conquer our thirst for economic growth and our ever-growing consumption of fossil fuels. We need to end industrial agricultural practices and forest clearing. While the populations of the West – with their high income levels and high fossil fuel consumption under capitalism – have created this problem, the South will be the first to suffer. There is a need then for redistribution from North to South. As Weston (2011) argues, the basis of that redistribution should be the massive ecological debt to be paid by the North to the South in the wake of the rape of the South by colonial powers.

This notion of the ecological debt stems from the historical claim that the industrialised West exploited the developing world, both enriching themselves and impoverishing developing countries. According to Acción Ecológica (2005), today's 'form of looting uses subtler methods' than in the past. These include 'the foreign debt promoted by the countries of the North; the promotion of the international market on terms which favour them; the flow of foreign investment; the privatisation of energy, communications, water, and the earth', et cetera. It is also argued that these policies 'are promoted by … the IMF, the World Bank and … the WTO which seek to dictate world economic policy in order to maintain this system of dominance'.

There are at least three reasons why markets cannot solve the problem of global warming. First, capitalism needs growth to survive; if that 'engine' is taken away capitalism will collapse. Second the pace of reform of the main market policy proposed – carbon pricing – is all too slow. The science is clear that urgent action is needed. A new 'shock doctrine', not to bring in neoliberalism as dissected by Naomi Klein (2007), but to get rid of it, is required. The ability of governments and other agencies to monitor and regulate adequately what is going on with respect to emissions is also to be doubted. Third, the source of denialism which is a truly major problem in addressing global warming is rooted in capitalism itself with its short term-ism, its focus on growth, and its inability to take adequate account of the 'externalities' it creates environmentally.

This lack of adequate mechanisms to internalise externalities means that any carbon pricing scheme will fail.

Any such scheme that allows the rich North to offset its emissions by buying relief in the South will spell problems for the South. The same is true of any attempts to go down the road of biofuels – which are already reducing the supply of food, as agricultural land that has previously been used to feed the peoples of the South is used to feed the motor vehicles of the North. As Goklany argues, 'Policies to increase production and use of biofuels retard the developing world's progress against reducing poverty levels and would exacerbate their burden of death and disease from the various diseases of poverty' (2011: 12). According to his analysis in 2010, 'the production of biofuels may have led to at least 192,000 additional deaths and 6.7 million additional lost DALYs'.

Perhaps most worrying is that there is currently no global body that has either the power or the will to come up with global solutions. The UN is weak and too often ignored by the rich Western nations. The rich West instead places its faith in the Bretton Woods financial organisations of the World Bank, the IMF and the WTO – all of which are controlled by the West and operate on neoliberal principles (see Chapter 4.) Such 'ownership' and ideology do not bode well for adequate solutions emerging from these sources. Such neoliberally driven bodies are unlikely to want to sound the death knell of neoliberalism.

A further concern at the level of global distribution is that currently the way in which emissions are calculated is biased against developing countries. This is because emissions from production processes are attributed to the producing country. This means, for example, that French people can increase their consumption of goods produced in China without any contribution being recorded for the emissions for France, while these emissions are attributed to the Chinese as the producers.

The impact of this 'transfer' is that the rich importing countries are made to look lesser villains – and vice versa for the poor exporting countries – than they otherwise would be in emitting carbon into the atmosphere. Of course this does not affect the overall global situation, but in geopolitical negotiations over climate change, it does alter the perception of the burden of damage and in turn of responsibility for action. It is the poor countries, which also have the major health problems currently, who need most support in addressing climate change. It is their health that will suffer most as global warming develops further. Any shift in the attribution of responsibility in the direction of the developing countries – which, in a neoliberal world run by neoliberal global institutions, are already politically weak – makes their situation and their bargaining powers yet weaker. From the perspective of global health, if there is to be any bias in favour of the rich or the poor, it ought to be in the latter direction.

It is troubling that the calculation of emissions is done in this way and there must be strong reason to believe it was deliberate on the part of those who devised this scheme. The key here lies in assessing who devised the Kyoto Agreement, since this way of attributing carbon emissions stems from that agreement. To a considerable extent it is no longer possible to deconstruct what happened in reaching that agreement, but what we do know is that it was hammered out by and large by developed countries.

Weston (2011) places the blame for the design of the Kyoto Protocol firmly on the US which, she argues, was 'in turn … heavily influenced by the fossil fuel and automobile industry interests'. She continues: 'The rich nations, it was argued by the US negotiators, should be allowed to buy their cuts from other countries, and to sell the gases they weren't producing to other nations; and that rich nations could buy nominal cuts from poor ones.' Having won the day in getting this agreement, the US then refused to sign!

South Africa, the World Bank and coal

What happens, in terms of the containment of global warming, when a neoliberal government is aided and abetted by a neoliberal global institution? In this example, the government is South Africa. The global institution is the World Bank.

The South African government is planning a massive increase in electricity generation by 2025. This is to be achieved through doubling its electricity generation capacity from coal-fired power stations. South Africa has an abundance of coal.

The World Bank has become heavily involved in assisting in the funding of the expansion of these coal-fired power stations. This was rumoured from 2008 onwards. Despite the protests of many civil society organisations, largely because of the impact on global warming, the largest World Bank loan ever in Africa – US$3.75 billion to Eskom, the South African parastatal – was announced in April 2010. This is, to say the least, somewhat paradoxical, given that the World Bank's Strategic Framework on Development and Climate Change argues that there is a need to act quickly on global warming. Further, it suggests that otherwise global warming could undo various recent development efforts, including attempts to achieve the United Nations' eight Millennium Development Goals for poverty reduction. Redman (2008) indicates, though, that this loan is not out of line with other World Bank actions, as the Bank's lending for coal, oil and gas has increased by more than 90 per cent from 2007. Its lending for coal alone went up two and a half times in that period.

This is noteworthy given that, first, the production and burning of coal is such a major emitter of carbon dioxide and, second, the World Bank is supposed to be the lead global organization in the fight to save the planet, and is thus an important player at the international global warming negotiating table.

We should also note that, during the period of apartheid, the World Bank lent $100 million to Eskom. These loans did nothing for black communities and some of the victims of apartheid have taken legal action against the banks that profited from these loans. It is also suggested by Bond (2010) that the World Bank co-authored the 1996 Growth, Employment and Redistribution (GEAR) programme, which signalled the end of any real post-apartheid attempt to redistribute income to the poor. That GEAR policy amounted to the endorsement of neoliberalism. It also resulted in black incomes subsequently falling below 1994 levels while white incomes grew by 24 per cent. Swilling (2010) argues that the loan gives the World Bank what it really wants and has never had before, a firm grip on the South African economy and influence over economic policy. In 2001, in a policy announcement, the World Bank stated that 'The Bank will focus on countries which demonstrate – through actions –

a credible intent to privatise and to liberalise ... liberalisation of power supply will be pursued through privatisations and the removal of legislative and commercial barriers to public/private partnerships' (quoted in Bond 2002: 318).

Going back to *The Lancet* paper on the health effects of global warming (Costello *et al.* 2009), it is very clear from the granting of this loan to South Africa for coal-generated electricity and in Redman's disclosure of the extent of the build-up of loans more generally from the World Bank for coal, oil and gas projects, that the Bank has no real interest, despite its posturing, in tackling global warming. Given its central global role in negotiations over climate change, the probability of any globally coherent policies emerging on global warming is currently zero.

Yet this – global warming – is the biggest threat to human health. It is especially countries such as South Africa which will suffer first and most, and it is the health of those in developing countries which is first and most at risk. The World Bank does not just watch on as a spectator, although if it did that would be a serious enough abrogation of its global responsibilities. In its dedication to the edicts of neoliberalism, it is adding fuel to the fire of global warming.

So what is the answer?

This I will address in more detail in the subsequent chapters, but it is clear there needs to be radical change in the way we organise our lives, our economies and our societies. The lifestyle of the rich West is unsustainable and has to be reined in and re-orientated if we are to do much if anything to protect the health of those in the developing world. They have not created the problem; the West has. It is the lives of people in the developing world, and their health, which will suffer first. The ecological debt needs to come into play. It is pay-back time.

Capitalism is dependent on economic growth. Yet the planet cannot be saved if we continue to expand our economies and our use of fossil fuels. There needs to be a new political economy. There is a case for investing as fast as we can in new technologies and for experiments with renewables. Even many of the most ardent supporters of renewables readily admit that they can only be a partial solution. The only debate here is how big a part.

So, as Weston (2011) states, the choice is between capitalism and the planet. Only one can survive.

PART IV / Solutions

The solutions in theory: communitarian claims

I have previously argued for a move away from an essentially 'utilitarian' health policy to communitarianism (Mooney 2009). Here I shall set out the idea of 'communitarian claims' as a basis for health policy, showing how this can first bring the community into the decision-making process; and second allow those disadvantaged people who, in Amartya Sen's words, 'have an inability to manage to desire adequately' (1992) to have access to better health and health care. This chapter forms the theoretical base for what follows in the rest of the book.

It is crucial, I believe, to shift the power base of health policy. Pivotal to what I have to say is the idea of health-care systems as social institutions, and of the social determinants of health as very much social – defined by and valued by the critically informed community, and allowed to vary according to different relevant cultural values. For example, in looking at inequalities in an African setting, income inequalities are poor proxies for power relations, as might be the case in some Western construct of class. The culturally appropriate power relations in Africa are often based, for example, on past colonial influences and experiences. The question then is how to determine the value bases or principles on which to operate in this territory.

Communitarianism

The philosophy behind the approach is that of communitarianism; the mechanisms are what I have previously dubbed communitarian claims (Mooney 2009). First let me spell out communitarianism.

The focus of communitarianism is public life and the community.

People are not, as in liberalism, free-floating atoms but rather social animals. Their being is composed in part by the community in which they exist; being in and of a community matters, and they take their identity partly from that. The community is not just a collectivity (although it is that); it is also valued in itself and is more than the sum of individual parts. The notion derived from neoclassical economics of individuals setting out to maximise their own individual utility (or preferences) is alien, at least as an iron law. The individual has an identity that is based in large part on being a member of a community, or more accurately a member of possibly several communities. Individuals do have autonomy, but the notion of community or social autonomy is strong. Lying behind communitarianism are such values as sharing and reciprocity. People are involved in community participation because their sense of identity, their security and their survival all spring from there. Such involvement is in a sense out of 'self-interest', but also out of a sense of 'community interest', and the two then merge.

The term 'community' is construed in many different ways. In health and health care, it is most likely to have a geographical reference, since health-care systems and population health issues tend to cover geographical locations. Such geographical areas, however, could be small – such as villages or towns – or could go all the way up to the nation state and beyond to the global community. They might also cover cultural or ethnic groupings, especially when these have specific (to them) constructs of health.

Citizenship is closely linked to communitarianism. An important distinction needs to be made between a consumer and a citizen. This is well exemplified by Macpherson:

> One can acquire and consume oneself, for one's own satisfaction or to show one's superiority to others … whereas the enjoyment and development of one's capacities is to be done for the most part in conjunction with others, in some relation of community. And it will not be doubted that the operation of participatory democracy would require a stronger sense of community than now prevails. (1977: 99–100)

In the literature the name most associated with citizenship is that of Marshall, who considered citizenship in

> three parts ... civil, political and social. The civil element is composed of the rights necessary for individual freedom ... the political element ... [involves] the right to participate in the exercise of political power ... the social element [is] the whole range from the right to a modicum of economic welfare and security to the right to share to the full in the social heritage and to live the life of a civilised being according to the standards prevailing in the society. (1950: 10)

Avineri and de-Shalit argue that 'communitarians conclude that, in order to justify the special obligations that we hold to members of our communities – families, nations, and so forth – one must attach some intrinsic (i.e. non-instrumental) value to the community' and that, as compared with any individualistic theory, communitarian theory 'better justifies obligations that are not universal but rather specific and particular, because these obligations are part of what constitutes the self' (1992: 3). This notion of community results in a different world view, particularly with respect to the idea of health care as a commodity. Commodified care, because to a very great extent an individualised 'entity', is foreign to communitarianism. Health-care systems become social institutions under a communitarian gaze, or at least they have a greater chance of becoming so.

It would be wrong to label the economist, philosopher and Nobel Laureate Amartya Sen a communitarian. However, in forming an overall assessment of an individual's interests, Sen suggests we need to consider not only the individual's own well-being but also what he calls her 'agency achievement and agency freedom', which are relative to goals that stretch beyond her personal well-being. In explaining agency Sen writes:

> A person as an agent need not be guided only by her own well-being, and agency achievement refers to the person's success in the pursuit of the totality of her considered goals and objectives. If a person aims at, say, the independence of her country, or the prosperity of her community, or some such general goal, her agency achievement would involve evaluation of states of affairs in the light of these objects, and not merely in the light of the extent to which those achievements would contribute to her own well-being. (1992: 56)

Sen is using the independence of her country and the prosperity of her community only as examples, but both as it happens fit with a communitarian outlook.

Trust can immediately be seen, in this discussion, as an important ingredient of communitarianism. In individualistic societies suspicion and distrust are more likely; and cohesion and participation less likely. While accepting that there is no one uniquely correct definition of communitarianism, there are however some key common elements in all interpretations. As compared with the universalism claimed by liberal philosophers for liberalism, at least in the form developed by Rawls (1971) in his theory of justice, communitarians see both justice and social values more generally as being embedded in a society. It follows that their conceptualisation and contextualisation are, or at least can be, particular to each society. That makes things messier – how do we allocate resources equitably across different countries or cultures if there is no common construct of equity? The Scandinavians, for example, would seem to place more weight on equity than the US does, both in their health-care systems and in society more generally. Within a country such as Australia with a substantial Indigenous population, trying to be 'fair' across two different cultures – Aboriginal and non-Aboriginal – is inevitably difficult. It is also the case that the construct of health is cultural, so dealing with some notion of equity – say, equal access for equal health need – is potentially problematic. Trying to find some fair way to allocate apples and pens to two groups who disagree about what is fair and who also attach different values to both apples and pens seems well nigh impossible! My solution to this problem later in this chapter is not perfect, but may help.

Wilkinson, if not explicitly from a communitarian perspective, offers this:

> [I]t is important to recognise that our emotional ability to identify with each other is broadening, if not deepening. Where once people apparently felt quite unaffected by the suffering of any but their nearest and dearest, it looks as if the boundaries of our moral universe have been expanding: our tendency to identify with each other is slowly spreading from family to class, from class to nation, and now, for some at least, to most of the human race. (2005: 296)

I would agree, but under neoliberalism the extent to which humanity is prepared to be humane – take the treatment of refugees, for example – is really quite limited.

The assumed universalism of liberalism in the context of health is questioned by Adams when she writes of: 'the idea of an equity of epistemology – about the way we theorise health and its causes – in international arenas' (2004: 3). She goes on to conclude that 'these concerns, cumulatively, point to ineffable areas of ethics in health and health equity' – basically, that we simply cannot find words to explain these phenomena.

Communitarianism thus has the advantage of having no pretensions to be a universalist philosophy, and can be country- and culture-specific. Of course, there can be no guarantee against communities being wicked, such as the community that was Nazi Germany. Communitarianism is only good if the community it draws on is good. The prospects for goodness, though, do seem greater in a community where individuals are more rather than less embedded. Here Dworkin (1989) suggests that in an integrated community 'everyone, of every conviction and economic level, has a personal stake ... in justice not only for himself but for everyone else as well'. Thus there are no guarantees of goodness, but the chances are higher.

Communitarians are very much concerned not only with the shape of society but also with the shaping of society. They do not believe that this can be left to individuals *qua* individuals. Two potentially important caveats need to be entered here. First, there will almost certainly have to be some efforts made to educate the citizenry, such that this shaping of the community is done on an informed basis. Second, depending on such factors as the homogeneity of the society and the extent of social solidarity, there is a risk that minority groups will not have their claims adequately recognised by the majority. That question, and whether to allow this within the community, needs to be debated and indeed resolved.

Levels of preferences

What is needed is to sort out how different sorts of preferences can be assessed. Take the example of chocolate. I have an 'impulse' preference for chocolate which means I occasionally indulge myself. At the same time I am into physical fitness and I recognize that over-indulging in chocolate is not good for me. So there is this second more reflective and longer-term level of preferences. What I am also postulating is that as a member of the community I might, together with other members of the community, come to a view that chocolate from a community perspective is harmful – and so we might as a community try to be less dependent on chocolate. So we have this third level of preferences. These are communitarian preferences.

We can note in passing that in 1970 Richard Titmuss published his book *The Gift Relationship*, which was about the supply of blood and what difference it might make if this were done voluntarily or commercially. He made the case for it being better to raise it voluntarily, writing: 'Altruism in giving to a stranger does not begin and end with blood donations. It may touch every aspect of life ... it is likely that a decline in the spirit of altruism in one sphere of human activities will be accompanied by similar changes in attitudes, motives and relationships elsewhere.' This is communitarianism at work.

Communitarian preferences, the preferences of citizens *qua* citizens, are normally ignored by economists. This is largely because the economics profession so seldom recognises people as citizens. But we do have preferences at that level. We do take pride in our country; we do want our society to be decent and fair. We have preferences for how our governments deal with asylum seekers, global warming, the treatment of the poor. We care about our institutions. For example, is the justice system just? We may value the fact that our health service is available to all even if that means we have to pay more in taxes for those less well off than ourselves.

Trying to grapple with these three levels of preferences is difficult. What follows concentrates on the 'new' level – that is, the communitarian preferences.

Communitarian claims

Twenty years ago John Broome suggested that in dealing with issues of fairness there is a need to separate the reasons why someone should receive some good or service into two categories, what he called 'claims' and other reasons (1991: 61). He went on to argue that the idea of a claim to a good means 'a duty owed to the candidate herself that she should have it'. Broome went on to argue that claims 'are the object of fairness'.

I have previously suggested moving Broome's concept of claims to make it more relevant to communitarianism. First I propose that 'communitarian claims' be a sub-set of claims more generally where this sub-set is the responsibility of the community to meet or address. Thus the duty in the case of communitarian claims is a duty owed by the community.

These claims are called communitarian claims because it is the community who decide what constitute claims and the weights to be attached to them. It is also considered that members of the community will see value for themselves in being involved in this process.

Having set this idea in motion I have come to realise that the word 'claim' is less than ideal in this context because in normal parlance it usually needs whoever is to benefit to exercise her claim – that is, an active role for the person who is to benefit from the claim.

> 'I claim' and 'you claim' is standard usage where this is shorthand for 'I claim on my behalf' and 'you claim on your behalf'. Here we the community determine how resources are allocated on the basis of how we the community determine first what constitute claims – what are deemed relevant criteria for allocating health-care resources – and how we the community see various different groups' or individuals' strengths of claims for the resources involved. It is our preferences, the community's preferences, for their claims, the various groups' claims, that determine how the resources are allocated. It is we the community who also decide what is relevant in identifying and weighting claims in terms of the characteristics of the different potential recipient groups and the community as a whole. (Mooney and Russell 2005)

What this means is that the values that are to determine how resources are allocated are those of the community. They determine the basis of claims and the weights to be attached to different claims.

Claims in practice

We can speculate about what might constitute claims and their weights. These might include age, socio-economic status, ethnicity, timing and distribution, rural/urban, availability of alternatives, with dependants/without dependants, whether recipients are 'contributors' or 'drains' on society, et cetera. Research is needed to establish these and it is assumed that they are likely to vary from one society to another.

One example (see Mooney 2010) of using claims with a citizens' jury came up with the following initial list of bases for claims. These are given in no particular order, but rather as they 'came up' for a specific, embedded group of citizens. Conceivably they will strike the reader as 'rough and ready', but the whole point here is to exemplify the dynamic process involved, and the kind of interchange within a particular community that can yield a result that the participants perceive as 'fair' and answering to their (communitarian) purpose.

- Poor health
- People who have had a raw deal
- Being poor
- Rural areas
- Elderly
- Children
- Aboriginality
- Overweight/obese
- Vulnerable/marginalised groups
- Poor access
- Feedback to the community
- Unemployed
- Mentally ill
- Chronic disease
- Prevention/health promotion.

There were in this instance thus many bases for claims, which is hardly surprising. The key ones were:

- Poor health
- Marginalised/vulnerable populations, especially Aboriginal people and mentally ill people
- Poor access for a range of reasons, but especially poverty and geographical – that is, rural location.

The sources of high or strong claims on resources can be summarised largely as disadvantage – with poverty, Aboriginality and mental illness being the factors where the health service involved might best devote its energies and resources.

With respect to the relative strengths of claims, poverty emerged as the strongest claim, ahead of both poor health and Aboriginality. The aggregation of claims was not possible but the strength of claims of poor, Aboriginal people, in poor health, would clearly be high.

Strengths of claims were also elicited from this jury. For poor people (average annual household income of $30,000) compared to rich (average $100,000) the weight was over 4. For poor health (life expectancy of 60) versus better health (life expectancy of 80) the ratio was 2:1. For Aboriginal versus non-Aboriginal the ratio was just under 2. Additional 'strengths of claims' established were 2:1 children to adults; 1.5:1 elderly to adults; and 1:1 men to women.

Conclusion

This chapter has sought to spell out the theoretical and conceptual underpinnings of my proposal for a new political economy of health. The key considerations here involve a shift in power to citizens; genuine participation of citizens in health and health-care planning; an emphasis on the community and in turn on communitarianism; and communitarian claims. The power shift is what really holds the key. Most fundamentally this involves the recognition that there are issues where it is critically informed people, citizens, who must be allowed to have their voice heard in what is their health-care system and their society.

13 / The solutions in health care

How to build on communitarian claims in health care

The previous chapter laid out the basis of how in theory a new health-care system might be devised. Here I want to look at possible solutions in more detail and in a more practical way. That cannot be prescriptive, and there is no universally 'right' way to organise health care. Indeed, given the social and cultural bases that this book has argued should underpin health-care organisations, these will inevitably and rightly assume different forms in different societies. Nonetheless, some key issues at a more practical level can be spelt out here.

A political economy of health care

The way to overcome the current problems in health-care systems is threefold: first, to get acceptance of the need for a debate about who exercises power over resource allocation in health care, and about who should exercise power at what levels; second, thereby to gain greater recognition that the issue is one of political economy; and third, to seek to influence the nature, funding, principles and priorities in this sector by shifting power to the citizenry. That means that health-care systems need to be seen much more as social institutions based on communitarian principles and with much more active participation of the citizenry in health services, or at least in setting the principles underlying such services.

There is also considerable merit in 'localising' decision making around local health problems and solutions. Clearly not all health-care decision making can take place in a local setting – not each locality of say a few thousand people can have a teaching hospital, for example. But many health and health-care problems are local, and to build upwards and move away from the top-down planning which is so common in health care is surely welcome. What is suggested here fosters such an approach.

The key is political economy. What I mean by that is that to move health-care systems to embrace what I would call social efficiency and social equity, two things are needed in policy analysis and health-care governance. First, there needs to be a clear recognition of where power lies in health-care decision making and, second, that power must be transferred to the community and society supposedly served by the health services.

The evidence for this argument, this strategy, is simple. Look at almost any health-care system (though I'll look at some that are different in the next three chapters) and what do we see? A goal of benefit (health?) maximisation? An equitable distribution of health-care resources? Doctors and other health-care staff trained and employed to pursue such objectives? Transparency to the public in how resources are allocated and by whom? No. And the big question that this book seeks to address is as simple. Why not?

Some of the case studies examined earlier give part of the answer and tell a different story from that which would emerge from social efficiency and equity. In South Africa, as indicated in Chapter 7, around half of the health-care 'spend' goes to the 16 per cent of the population in the private schemes, yet these are the people who are already better off economically – read much better off – and considerably healthier than the others. The others – the poor, and the majority of very poor who make up the other 84 per cent, then have to rely on the other half of the spend. Thus the great bulk of South Africans who use only the public health services, but who are poor and thus carry a much higher burden of disease, get only about one sixth of the spend per capita. In no language can that be termed efficient or equitable. We have here a classic case of Bob Evans's (1997) linking of the rich and powerful in the private sector with the willing connivance of the doctors to ensure that their health is looked after; that they only pay for their own health to be looked after; and that they avoid having to pay mightily through taxes to ensure that the health of others is looked after according to the same standards as their own. It then follows that the doctors earn good money serving the wishes and the health of the rich, which is financially and emotionally preferable to having to deal with the poor in the townships.

One only needs to look at the efforts of the private sector medical schemes in South Africa to protect their patch and ward off a national health insurance scheme to see how vulnerable the social objectives of efficiency and equity are to the leverage of organisations that serve those with economic power.

The major shift needed in practice is to change the way in which health services are governed, starting with the idea of treating them not only as social institutions but wherever possible as local institutions – there to serve the public and to be driven by the values of the community which the services are supposed to be serving.

There also needs to be an increase in transparency, particularly around priority setting – currently so shrouded in confusion and uncertainty that it becomes well-nigh impossible for anyone to ascertain how or why priorities are set as they are. Indeed, the situation is so bad in many health-care systems that there often appears to be no explicit system of priority setting, or that what passes for priority setting is little more than wish listing.

It is this lack of an explicit, rational, informed priority-setting system that I see as one reason for the malaise in modern-day health-care systems. The much-applauded Oregon health-care priority-setting system (Dixon and Welch 1991) was a pale imitation of what is needed. Initially it sought to rank interventions in terms of both benefits and costs (which is good) although later costs were dropped for political reasons. This was rather odd since the reason why priority setting is needed is because there has to be some limit on spending, and hence on costs. The (US-based) Oregon approach also failed to recognise that there is a need to look at priority setting in terms of how many interventions, and for whom.

A constitution for health care

Yet more explicitly, health services need to be underpinned by a constitution set by the citizenry through communitarian claims. Such a constitution is really a set of principles or values on which to base the organisation and running of health services. While many countries have motherhood statements of their visions and goals, few that I am aware of are based on well-thought-out principles as set by the society in any way directly. It is often the case that health services do have goals or objectives and that is fine, although seldom are these based on the views of the community. To get the community more involved in such goal setting would be good, but the idea of a constitution is somewhat different.

The economist Vanberg (1994) argues that organisations can be of three types: they can be exchange- or market-based; they can be goal-orientated; or they can be based on a constitutional paradigm. It is clear that most health-care systems are market-based (or draw heavily on the market ideology of consequentialism) or goal-orientated – and thus also essentially consequentialist or outcome-focused. Few, as far as I can see, are based on a set of principles, however derived, let alone one issuing directly from the community.

Yet what is a health-care system but an organisation that is there to deliver health care to some community or society, which pitches in through taxation or insurance premiums and/or direct payments for the service – and, crucially, for the service to be there if and when they need it. It would seem to matter to the community how the services are paid, and there are few existing health services that do not involve some form of cross-subsidisation – not always from rich to poor but sometimes, as with private health insurance, from rich (well) to rich (sick). How do the rules regarding such cross-subsidisation get drawn up? In most instances this is not at all clear.

Again, since no health service does or can aim to provide all health care for all, there are then questions of eligibility for membership, and who decides that. And for those members, what rules govern how still-limited resources are allocated to different members – and who decides on these rules? The health service will have to decide 'its' priorities, which might be across different diseases, different age or ethnic groups, or different disease groups. How much to cure? To prevention? To palliative care?

So what I am advocating for health-care systems is that they adopt a social institutional ethos which is built on a constitution, while this in turn is based on the values of the population the system is to serve. What might this entail? Vanberg describes it thus:

> From a constitutional perspective, the essential definitional attribute of an organisation is that a group of persons, for whatever interests or goals, submit with some of their resources to certain constitutional constraints, to a set of common rules, including rules for changing rules. That is, not some imputed common interest or goal, but a common constitution is the essential basis of an organisation, the link that ties its members together. (1994: 138)

Perhaps even more important is the point that Vanberg makes about the customers of a firm who 'typically are not members of the organisation and have no constitutional right to be included in the firm's decision-making process' (1994: 139). In health care currently 'customers' or 'consumers' clearly have 'no constitutional right to be included in the firm's decision-making process'.

In health care in recent years the language of the market has come in quite strongly; we now have providers, business plans, consumers and customers. In health-care debates, the word patient is dismissed as being too passive or compliant. That may be true, but to switch to customers and consumers leaves the patients solely on the demand side of the market. Given the nature of the demand here, which is very individualistic and often based on major uncertainty, the potential for countervailing power in the health-care market is minimal. The supply side dominates, which would not matter if it could be left to the politicians to ensure that the supply side – what is made available – reflected the wishes of the community. That seldom happens; to assume that it would is to ignore the power of the medical profession and the medical associations in health-care planning. To make this a reality in terms of the constitution, I would argue for citizens' juries – mentioned earlier and discussed further below – as a form of deliberative democracy.

To get the citizenry heavily involved in health-care planning is not practical. Athenian democracy has its appeal but the opportunity costs are just too high. As indicated, I propose that we devise and adopt a set of principles for social choice – a 'constitution' – for health services. This involves a set of principles on which policy and actions might be based: such as equity, how important it is and how it might be defined. Is there to be concern only with horizontal equity, the equal treatment of equals, or also vertical equity and the unequal but equitable treatment of unequals? A constitution might cover issues of respect for individual autonomy, of ensuring the freedom of individuals to refuse treatment, of the extent to which only outcomes matter or whether processes (such as decision making *per se*) are also to be valued. It might even state in which contexts in public health the community's preferences should count, and when valuation issues might be left to the experts.

The idea of stepping back and thinking through the principles on which societies seek to build their health services is a simple one. Questions of the appropriateness of health care, of evidence bases, of the measurement of health outcomes – all potentially laudable – cannot be satisfactorily nor comprehensively addressed until there is clarity with respect to the values that do and should drive the health-care system. That set of values in my view has to come from the community.

What is possible is to bring critically informed public preferences into health-service decision making without all the complexities and costs of Athenian democracy. This involves using the community voice to establish the underpinning values and leaving the 'experts' to operationalise the constitution.

Looking to health services as social institutions means that they become more akin to social services, where the inputs are not simply the resources of the health services but involve also the resources of the citizens. This is most obvious at the level of the patient and his or her carers in the community. Citizens, however, can also be involved as a resource in health care in the sense of their time and effort in offering their informed preferences for the procedural foundations of health care – in other words, its constitution.

Freedman (nd) agrees that we need to think of a health-care system as a social institution and not just as a way of delivering health. Her concern in making this point is with the Millennium Development Goals (MDGs). She suggests that the framing of these goals

> invites a technocratic, largely top-down approach with a familiar sequence of steps: determine the primary causes of the MDG diseases/ conditions; measure the incidence and prevalence; identify the medical interventions to prevent or treat these causes; determine the most cost-effective delivery systems for those interventions; calculate the costs; advocate for 'political will' to get the job done. (*Ibid.*:1)

Lucy Gilson argues neatly that health systems 'are not only producers of health and health care, but they are also purveyors of a wider set of societal norms and values' (2003: 1461). I would agree that they are thus social institutions which ought to be based on society's values. It is not enough to see health-care systems as delivering health in some purely mechanical way, as in some factory process. The population served are not simply 'passive' consumers. They are part of the process of production of health care, inevitably so, though this is so often forgotten. They are also the society that is dependent on its social institutions to thrive as a society, and the health-care system is one such social institution among many – the education system, the courts, the market and so on. They can be critical in how a society develops or fails to develop.

One such example is the development of National Health Insurance (NHI) in South Africa (where I am writing this part of the book in August 2011), for which a Green Paper has just been published (Department of Health 2011). Clearly such an NHI is designed to deliver health to the South African people. My argument is that it is more than that. It is or will be a social institution that can help to build a more united country and show the way to create other socially uniting institutions in this deeply fractured country. What will be interesting to observe is how the debate on South Africa's NHI develops, and whether it is restricted to the delivery of health or branches out into concerns about building social institutions, which in turn can help to lead to a more united and decent society. We must wait and see.

Thus in South Africa as elsewhere, the way of looking at health-care systems advocated here is seeking to set such systems within a communitarian framework. That can allow *inter alia* a more cohesive society to emerge. Such cohesion or solidarity can act as an antidote to the individualism promulgated by neoliberalism and in turn, as the literature on the social determinants of health suggests, can act positively on population health. It also encourages greater participation in society, which becomes more caring since social isolation is reduced and people are literally more likely to know and communicate with their neighbours.

What this endorses is the need in various discussions and planning exercises about health-care resource allocation to think in terms not just of goals or objectives, but to look to the principles that might underpin such plans. Too often such value considerations are omitted and planning becomes almost wholly a technocratic exercise. An example is how primary health care is discussed in the South African Green Paper on the NHI (Department of Health 2011). The emphasis of the thinking is almost wholly on how to do it, and too little on the value base on which these services might be based. Is equity an underlying principle? If so, how is that to be defined? Is transparency in decision making in public health care an issue? How will that be defined – and transparency about what, to whom? In other words, what is to be the constitution for South African public health care?

These questions need to be asked, even if answering them is difficult. Currently, in most health-care planning they are passed by and the focus is too often narrowly defined technocratic goals. These questions also often require answers regarding the longer term, often longer than politicians or health service decision makers will be around. Those who will be around long-term are the citizens served by these health services. These are the people who can provide what Stephen Jan (2003) calls 'credible commitment' to the social institution that is health care.

Citizens' juries

There are a number of different forms of deliberative democracy which might serve to obtain at least some approximation to communitarian values, and in turn help with establishing communitarian claims. My preferred approach is that of citizens' juries (Mooney and Blackwell 2004). These seek to bring a representative cross-section of the community together, usually through a process of random selection of citizens; have a group of experts present relevant information to them; and give them the opportunity to question the experts. The jury is then left to deliberate on what they have learned and come to some consensus on matters that usually relate to the values or principles they want their health services based on, and the priorities they want that health service to pursue. It is emphasised throughout that they are there as citizens representing the community, and that they face real resource constraints and hence the need to prioritise. It is of course possible to use such juries for other purposes, but my experience suggests that members of juries will switch off if they feel they are being asked to form judgements about issues that they believe are not in their province. They will quickly realise, for example, that issues around, say, choice of medicines for heart disease are beyond their capabilities, and that there are other people who are much better placed to form such judgements. They do tend to agree, however (perhaps not surprisingly), that a basic principle of any health service should be that citizens should set the principles and broad priorities! It is also the case that with respect to communitarian claims, values and priorities are all that are needed from them.

It remains the case that as of now there is no agreement as to what form of deliberative democracy is best. Others advocate the use of focus groups, opinion polls and conjoint analysis. What is best may well vary depending on the purpose of the exercise. Thus:

> In the literature there is little discussion on what approach to use in eliciting community preferences. Is the intention to obtain community values by aggregating the preferences of individuals concerned for themselves? Or by asking individuals to put themselves in the position of planners acting on behalf of a community such as, say, the Perth community or the Australian community? Or are community values best discovered by allowing a communal discourse that gradually reveals a consensus? Each approach is likely to reveal a different set of community preferences. The usefulness of each approach will be partly dependent on what kind of decision making the results are intended to guide. (Mooney and Blackwell 2004)

What is sought in eliciting community values is a method that gets us as near as we can to critically informed, randomly selected, citizens' values on the basis of some time spent reflecting together and acknowledging that there are resource constraints that health services face. Citizens' juries seem to fit the bill, but if other methods might prove better for eliciting values and claims, then let's use them. I have not found anything better so far.

There is more to this question of citizen engagement than simply eliciting values through citizens' juries or some other form of deliberative democracy. The more fundamental issue, beyond such elicitation, is getting citizens involved more generally, having them participate in community and social activities and in decision making that affects their lives. The emphasis in this book is getting citizens involved in health-care decision making and in other health-enhancing activities, but the essence of what is involved here is participation in the community and its various institutions. That can lead up to fostering and strengthening social institutions and in turn bolstering democracy. This takes the whole notion of participatory democracy to a different level, where governance issues are not just instrumental but are valued in their own right (Kashefi and Mort 2004).

These processes need to be seen by the citizens as 'genuine', however, otherwise cynicism will kill such exercises. There are all too many examples of token 'consultation' with the public in health-care planning (Glasner 2001). I have seen signs of this in a minority of those citizens that I have engaged with in citizens' juries. Most, however, have responded enthusiastically to such citizen engagement. They like being citizens and being given information that they can act upon to express responsibly their values in the belief that they can make a difference this way – to themselves, yes, but more importantly to the community. Kashefi and Mort (2004) indicate that what they call 'incidental consultations' can breed cynicism and be perceived as 'social control disguised as democratic emancipation'.

The goal of these exercises is clear. We want to establish for citizens what they see as justified claims over health-care resources. These may be related to efficiency considerations (for example, mental illness as a priority) or equity concerns (more resources for remote areas) or organisational issues (transparency in decision making).

Conclusion

While I am an advocate of citizens' juries and would want all health services to set up a family of these, I do not want any reader to feel that in rejecting these they thereby reject the whole idea of communitarianism, communitarian claims and the notion of health services as social institutions. They are but one means of getting to that 'citizens' constitution' and making the voice of citizens as a community heard in their health service. That is the key. That is how to fix the malaise of health-care systems.

14 / The solutions in society more generally

The end of neoliberalism?

The best outcome in terms of bringing about real change would be to see an end to neoliberalism. So many of the problems that beset societies today and their populations' health can be placed at its door. In chapters 15, 16 and 17 I will draw attention to Kerala, Cuba and Venezuela as three countries or regions of the world with ways of running their economies that have shown how better health can emerge in the wake of a local community focus. That I believe is the way to go.

Clearly not all countries will be able to throw off neoliberalism or to do so quickly, but it is still possible to think through on the basis of what we know of the social determinants of health what changes might be made in various countries to provide a better economic and social environment for the fostering of population health.

Some principles

Let me start with some broad principles and then go into more detail. In devising a strategy for the health of the nation, the key must be to build a society based on four key principles:

1 The elimination of poverty.
2 Greater equality not only in terms of income but in terms of power.
3 Greater participation and a stronger, thicker form of democracy.
4 A greater sense of community and of belonging.

Let me look at poverty and inequality together. While different phenomena, in policy terms they are closely linked. Poverty is a killer. There is no doubting that, and while there can be claims that it has been reduced globally and in various nation states, it continues strongly in too many places. Gadaffi was roundly condemned for turning on his people in Libya, with the result that many died. Yet not tackling poverty in any rich Western country is no less of a killer. The condemnation does not so readily follow, however. It should. Is the emotional distance we have from death by poverty a bit like the distance (from the brutal fact of killing) gained via the use of drones by the US military in Afghanistan and Pakistan? The point is made vividly by Wilkinson:

> We are used to feeling indignation at the human rights abuses in countries where people are imprisoned without trial, are tortured, or simply disappear, but health inequalities exact a much greater toll. What would we think of a ruthless government that arbitrarily imprisoned all less well-off people for a number of years equal to the average shortening of life suffered by the less privileged in our own societies? Given that higher deaths rates are more like arbitrary execution than imprisonment, perhaps we should liken the injustice of health inequalities to that of a government that executed a significant proportion of its population each year without cause. (2005: 18)

One of the keys to bringing about changes in poverty and inequality is taxation. Tax can do a number of things. First, it can help to reduce poverty. In fact I can see no other simple, quick way to do so. Taxation needs to be substantial in terms of the tax take moving the size of the public sector to say 50 per cent of GDP. This is a bit above where Scandinavian countries currently are. It would mean substantial tax increases in a number of countries.

It is not just a question of raising taxes but of taking the opportunity to ensure that the increases are progressive. There is a lot wrong with conventional economics but some aspects of it – those that have a ring of truth or common sense to them – can be useful. One is the mouthful of the 'diminishing marginal utility of income'. That just means that for every extra dollar someone has of income, the extra benefit or utility that person gets decreases.

So taking $100 in tax from a poor person hurts that person more than taking it from a rich person. But what if we take from the rich and give to the poor? So progressive taxation – the rich not only pay more taxation than the poor but they pay proportionally more – seems not only fair but does most for redistribution and hence for reducing inequality.

The other issue here is this. If someone is poor and his neighbours pass the hat round to help him out, everyone gets a good feeling. The poor man is financially better off. The richer givers get warm glows knowing they have helped a neighbour in trouble. This compassion or altruism has been described as the reason for taxation. Oliver Wendell Holmes suggested: 'Tax is what we pay for a civilised society.' And the Joly Report on taxation for the EU argued:

> Mobilisation of domestic resources for development through efficient and fair tax systems is crucial for sustainable growth, reducing aid dependency, poverty reduction, good governance and state building, including the provision of public services required to achieve the Millennium Development Goals (MDGs). Efficient and fair tax systems are integral to democracy, promote state legitimacy and strengthen the social contract and accountability between government and citizens. (Council of the European Union 2010)

Social exclusion or social isolation, issues around social support, and the nature and quality of housing are all issues that affect population health. Most fundamentally, however, these are issues that are driven by poverty and inequality. If poverty were eliminated and inequality reduced this would bring in its wake major improvements in these other social determinants of ill-health. The need for a rise in communitarianism – or social cohesion, social capital, solidarity – is clear. These all serve to break down the crass individualism of neoliberalism and in turn promote better population health.

The growth fetishism of neoliberalism is just that; a fetishism which defies any logic outside of neoliberalism. If it were the case that the infamous trickle-down did occur, then there might be some justification for the pursuit of growth, but the evidence on trickle-down's existence is just not there (as I discussed in Chapter 7 on South Africa).

Power and values

Crucially, the issues being discussed here relate to power, who holds it and how it is distributed. It is perhaps better to see this in terms of what amounts to the converse: being subjected to power, or loss of autonomy, which has a deleterious effect on health.

Here is the need to see such autonomy in the future in terms not of individual autonomy but of social or community autonomy, and in turn as a class issue. Issues of inequality of income have been the main focus of the literature in the social determinants of health and in largely descriptive terms. The social epidemiological analyses tend to see income inequalities as the cause of health problems rather than the symptoms. This in turn leads to a view that policy should aim at reducing income inequality. In doing that we need to recognise the point made by Navarro (2011): 'It is not inequalities that kill people. It is the people who produce and reproduce inequalities through their public and private interventions that kill people.'

Addressing inequality of income will help. I am not denying that. But a useful parallel may be found in the Australian example in Chapter 8 of victim blaming in obesity policy – rather than looking at and to the systemic issues regarding why people are driven to eat badly. Related is the question of what the economic system is doing or failing to do to create a climate where good eating is a socially responsible issue as interpreted by the community, and where the production, distribution and marketing of food are also driven by the interests and values of the community.

Being sucked into individualism is to be avoided, as that can take us away from seeing this as a question of the power structure in society. Similarly railing against the power of industrial barons is to miss the target; they cannot be categorised as victims in a neoliberal society, but they have little capacity to change their own behaviour. It is the system which gives them their power. It is the system that needs to change or be changed.

So what am I advocating here? It is summed up by Stefano Zamagni (nd) who writes:

> There is a difference between a situation where it is agreed that everyone pursues his own end (as in capitalistic enterprises) and a situation

where there is a common end to be shared. It is the same difference between a common good and a (local) public good. In the first case, the individual benefit deriving from it cannot be separated from the benefit that others enjoy from it too. In other words, individual interest is served together with others' interests, not against them, as with private good, or apart from them, as with a public good. In brief, while public is opposed to private, common is opposed to "own". Common is what is neither only your own, nor what is indistinctly everyone's.

That makes a lot of sense to me. As does Zamagni's further point:

> What is the economically significant consequence of this distinction? When the 'common' aspect of an action is limited to the means, the problem to be solved is the coordination of the actions of many subjects. On the other hand, when the 'common' aspect of an action goes beyond the means, then the problem to be solved is how to create cooperation.

My advocacy for an emphasis on social values that move us away from individual values and interests can be seen as threatening to those steeped in the individualism of the Western world. This individualism is deeply ingrained, so deeply in fact that autonomy is almost always interpreted as related to the freedom of the individual. The notion of community or social autonomy or freedom can appear to be an oxymoron. It is about giving power to the community, but fundamentally moving to a situation where it is the wish of individuals as members of a community to want the community to have such power.

This is not a plea for uniformity or a loss of individuality at that level. As Pascal (nd) wrote: 'Uniformity without diversity is useless to others; diversity without uniformity is ruinous for us. The one is harmful outwardly; the other inwardly.' It is the latter – the diversity without uniformity – that is the key to my argument here. Individuals as free-floating atoms can be free to 'do their own thing', to exercise their freedom of choice in the market place, to exercise the beloved consumer sovereignty of the neoclassical economist. But such freedom of diversity is a chimera. It is what Hegel railed against and Joan Robinson argued was a myth in capitalist societies. Without uniformity, without some common purpose within social groupings or communities, this neoliberal 'freedom' fails – and on three counts. First, in the market place it cannot be exercised by the vast majority of the world's population because they are poor; second, individuals qua individuals are largely powerless; and third, the 'community' strength that matters here is class, and that is missing or denied under neoliberalism. These are economic issues in the first place, and need to be seen as such. They also mean that a class interpretation must be adopted.

The question of what to do when consumer sovereignty fails is critical. Joan Robinson, one of the most eminent economists of the twentieth century, argues in a more general context that '[n]o-one who has lived in the capitalist world is deceived by the pretence that the market system ensures consumers' sovereignty'.

> The true moral to be drawn from capitalist experience is that production will never be responsive to consumer needs as long as the initiative lies with the producer. Even within capitalism consumers are beginning to organise to defend themselves. In a planned economy the best hope seems to be to develop a class of functionaries, playing the role of wholesale dealers, whose career and self-respect depend upon satisfying the consumer. They could keep in touch with demand through the shops; market research which in the capitalist world is directed to finding out how to bamboozle the housewife could be directed to discovering what she really needs; design and quality could be imposed upon manufacturing enterprises and the product mix settled by placing orders in such a way as to hold a balance between economies of scale and variety of tastes. (1972: 274)

Social institutions and compassion

It is worth recognising the contribution that the philosopher Hegel made to this debate as the nineteenth century was getting under way (Muller 2003: 157). Apart from anything else, we can at least acknowledge that this is by no means a new debate! Muller writes of Hegel:

> The pressures of competition ... gave market societies an outward thrust. The search for markets in which to sell these products for which supply now exceeded demand led entrepreneurs to push on into areas that were relatively backward economically, both internally and beyond the nation's borders.... Hegel recognised (as Adam Smith had not) that entrepreneurs were a major force in the expansion of the imagined wants of consumers ... the market did not just satisfy wants, it created them. (*Ibid.*)

What is yet more relevant in the context of this chapter, and in this book more generally, is the importance that Hegel attached to the state and in turn to social institutions. Hegel would have viewed neoliberals as being slaves to their passions. His view of freedom was very different and was grounded in the establishment of social institutions which were based in the 'local' culture and were thereby able to persuade people into good social habits. He saw the idea of social duties as enhancing freedom. He stated: 'In an ethical community, it is easy to say what someone must do and what the duties are which he has to fulfil in order to be virtuous. He must simply do what is prescribed, expressly stated, and known to him within his situation' (Hegel 1820: 150). In his conceptualisation of freedom, Hegel emphasised the crucial role of institutions 'so that self-conscious individuals could become more aware of the meaning of the institutions in which they participated – a step towards feeling at home in these institutions' (Muller 2003: 150).

This is all very different from the notion of market freedoms. Crucially, while it might be difficult for some readers to agree with this idea of freedom at the level of the individual *qua* individual, if we look at this through the eyes of a community then this notion of freedom does seem to be more acceptable. It is much easier to see it as being part of community life and in turn community freedom. This is apparent at the level of both duties to the community and duties by the community, a form of reciprocal agreement that for example is present in many Indigenous communities.

Social institutions matter. It is important that we as citizens of our own countries but also citizens of the world 'feel at home' in our institutions and that participation in social institutions, as integral parts of the state, is encouraged. There is further a need to defend our social institutions and, most fundamentally, to recognise the importance of, and in turn celebrate, the institution of community autonomy. A sense of belonging counts.

The social institutions that are health care, public health and health policy need more often to be recognised as valuable in their own right. Societies do value them for the health and other outcomes they produce, as conventional health economics implies; but these institutions *per se* can also be valued as contributing to a better, more decent society. They also need to be valued in more direct Hegelian terms as providing pillars (along with other social institutions) to protect the state, not least from being overrun by the forces of the neoliberal market place.

Moving away from the crass individualism of neoliberalism to a greater community focus will lead to the prospects of a more compassionate society. Where people see themselves as members of a community, they are more likely to be involved in reciprocity with other members and be concerned about issues of mutuality and trust than if they are individuals with fewer social ties. While these traits in a society cannot guarantee that it or its citizens will be more compassionate, where there is a commitment to one's community, the soil is likely to be more fertile; in turn compassion to others in that community may be more prevalent. The question of social compassion is yet more likely to occur in some sectors of the social fabric than others, with health care and public health looking to be better candidates for the presence of caring and compassion than, say, energy policy or transport. There are in many societies greater concerns with the health of others and/or the access to health care of others than is present in, say, the education of others. It is then possible to hypothesise that societies which are more communitarian in nature, such as the Scandinavian countries, will tend to be more concerned to protect the weak such as the sick and to see a social role for this protection (Juul Jensen 1987). That would in turn suggest a larger public sector, higher taxes and possibly more progressive taxation systems. It is difficult to measure compassion and even more so to measure differences in levels of compassion between different societies, but a case can be made for the characteristics listed above as being proxy measures of compassion.

Compassion without power, however, may not result in any significant differences in a society's overall policies towards vulnerable or disadvantaged people. It can be difficult for ordinary citizens to convey to those in power a desire to see a more compassionate society or a more compassionate workplace or a more caring school environment. The ruling ideology may be lacking in altruism or compassion, and often it is that which shapes social attitudes rather than the compassionate community persuading those in power to act compassionately.

The work of Martha Nussbaum on compassion, especially public compassion, is relevant. She asks:

> [W]hat would a compassionate society look like? Given that there is reason to think that compassion gives public morality essential elements of ethical vision without which any public culture is dangerously root less and hollow, how can we make this compassion do the best work it can in connection with liberal and democratic institutions?

And this is part of her answer:

> The insights of an appropriate compassion may be embodied in the structure of just institutions, so that we will not need to rely on perfectly compassionate citizens. This idea is used both by Smith (with his idea of the compassion of the 'judicious spectator') and by Rawls, who creates an artificial model of an appropriately constrained benevolence via the Original Position. This ideal of moral benevolence is the lens through which we see how institutions and basic political principles should be designed. (Nussbaum 2001: 403)

Thus Nussbaum argues that there are many different ways in which compassion might be built into our institutions. She does not, however, go so far as to argue that we can leave all of this to our institutions. Instead she suggests that we must 'rely on compassionate individuals to keep essential political insights alive and before our eyes' (Nussbaum 2001: 404). For her, the relationship between compassion and social institutions is 'a two-way street: compassionate individuals construct institutions that embody what they imagine; and institutions, in turn, influence the development of compassion in individuals' (2001: 405).

Hegel writes that 'it is of the utmost importance that the masses should be organised, because only [by] so do[ing do] they become mighty and powerful. Otherwise they are nothing but a heap, an aggregate of atomic units. Only when the particular associations are organised members of the state are they possessed of legitimate power' (quoted in Avineri 1974: 166). If the poor are not organised into some communal grouping, thereby giving themselves power, as individuals they will lose their autonomy. Community autonomy for the poor, but also for societies in general, matters. It is best achieved through institutionalising it.

PART V

How things might get better

15 / Kerala: community participation

Kerala's health

The case of Kerala, the state in the south-west of India, demonstrates both how to get the community involved and what the impact of that can be on both population health and the distribution of health.

India overall has very poor health, with an average expectation of life at birth of less than 62 years. It remains a poor country but currently, under the influence of neoliberal thinking and public policy, it is experiencing very rapid economic growth. A key question for health-policy makers in India might be: how best in this time of boom might the Indian population, as a whole, experience betterment in their health status?

Relevant to this question is the experience of the Indian state of Kerala (Narayana 2007). If it were possible for the rest of India to 'invest' in being like Kerala, this would lead to an estimated increase in years of life in India of approximately 11 billion. This is based on the simple calculation that there are 1.1 billion people in India and Kerala has an expectation of life at birth which is about 10 years higher than the rest of India.

At least part of the reason for this difference in Keralan health is historical and as such cannot be transferred to other parts of India (Narayana 2007). It was, for example, the first state in the world to elect democratically a communist government. Land ownership is such that over 90 per cent of Keralans own the land on which their home stands. Literacy among men is high compared to the rest of India (91 per cent compared with 52 per cent). For women the difference is yet greater: 86 per cent and 19 per cent respectively. But lessons can be learned from the nature of Keralan society that have had a bearing on its good health status and which may be applicable elsewhere.

Dreze and Sen argue that

> the contrast between [the two Indian states of] Uttar Pradesh [with an expectation of life at birth below the Indian average] and Kerala ... points to the special importance of a particular type of public action: the political organisation of deprived sections of the society. In Kerala, informed political activism, building partly on the achievement of mass literacy, has played a crucial role in the reduction of social inequalities based on caste, gender, and (to some extent) class. Political organisation has also been important in enabling disadvantaged groups to take an active part in the general processes of economic development, public action, and social change ... the concentration of political power in the hands of privileged sections of the society has contributed, perhaps more than anything else, to a severe neglect of the basic needs of disadvantaged groups.

This emphasis on public participation as the road to population health is again stressed by Sen in his *Development as Freedom*, where he writes that

> the general enhancement of political and civil freedoms is central to the process of development itself. The relevant freedoms include the liberty of acting as citizens who matter and whose voices count, rather than living as well-fed, well-clothed and well-entertained vassals. The instrumental role of democracy and human rights, important as it undoubtedly is, has to be distinguished from its constitutive importance. (1999: 288)

This public participation has been fostered through self-help groups (SHGs), which as Narayana remarks have 'taken some innovative forms':

> In Kerala, a new dimension was added to the SHG movement by the decentralisation of governance since 1996. The *panchayats*, or local self-government institutions, have begun sponsoring the SHGs (called *Kudumbasree*), largely of women, to channel poverty alleviation scheme funds. Almost every village now has a large number of *Kudumbasree* units. (Narayana 2007)

Why so good?

Much has been written of Kerala and its good health, although quite why its health is so good as compared to the other Indian states is not always clear. There are also concerns that some of that better health is being lost. Narayana (2007) provides perhaps the best summary of recent trends: 'low mortality, high morbidity, and high utilisation of private care summarise the story of health care in Kerala', and he adds that the use of private care has placed 'a heavy burden on the poorer segments of the population.' He also suggests that 'The large unorganized sector – farming, household manufacturing, and services – provides no financial protection against the cost of illness.' Yet the health of the people of Kerala is relatively good compared to the rest of India. It would seem we have to look elsewhere than health care for an explanation for that good health.

There is a history going back to the nineteenth century that is relevant to Kerala's reputation as a healthy state. Its maharajahs at that time were involved in developing public health programmes and later there was substantial investment in the training of nurses and doctors and the development of a network of hospitals. Of late, there appears to have been some slippage, with malaria re-emerging and new diseases becoming more prevalent – cancer, heart disease, hypertension and arthritis (Elamon *et al.* 2004). In the early 1990s, it was felt that there were still too many people who did not have access to clean water or latrines, while private-sector health was expanding, using expensive equipment for the few. There was then a recognition that something needed to be done.

That something emerged as the Kerala People's Campaign for Democratic Decentralization in 1996, which 'created a setting in which health activists could attempt to respond to the Kerala health sector crisis.' The state-level response was to allocate 35–40 per cent of the budget of the State Planning Board to local government units from 1997 to 2002, in a very real effort to stimulate local participation in planning services according to local preferences. This led to the preparation of local development reports for nearly 1,000 villages across Kerala. These set local priorities for which committees were established to determine how to proceed with their implementation. General guidelines were provided by the state but local councils were left with considerable autonomy in how to allocate the resources they were given. Health attracted between 13 and 15 per cent of the total. In three years (1997/8 to

1999/2000) over 47,000 health projects were implemented. These covered a wide range of actions that included latrine construction, nutrition, public health care, hospital equipment and burial grounds.

What this reflects at a more general level, as Mukherjee-Reed (2011) explains, is that in Kerala there is a 'history of mobilisations from above and below and synergies between "state" and "civil society" [that] have resulted in a culture of collective social experimentation which is quite unique'.

Some vignettes in Kerala

Given the importance of decentralised local decision making, the quite astonishing range of health-related activities and the desire to promote this diversity to accommodate local preferences and build community strengths, what I want to do in the rest of the chapter is to highlight a few 'local' examples which give some sense or flavour of what is a quite remarkable demonstration of local community autonomy at work.

Women and food security

Mukherjee-Reed (2011) tells of how Keralan women historically have been better off in terms of literacy, health care and maternity care than their counterparts elsewhere in India. It has been the case, however, that what he calls their 'social positioning or public participation' has lagged behind. This is changing, as '50 per cent of the seats in Kerala's local body elections are [being] reserved for women'.

He goes on to tell how women are coming together in large numbers – 250,000 throughout Kerala – to farm collectively, producing first for their own families but also to sell the surplus to the market. 'The idea is to increase the participation of women in agriculture, and in particular, to ensure that women, as producers, have control over the production, distribution and consumption of food.' Many, but not all, have experience of farming in the past but at that time led often rather isolated lives. Now they have a real sense of solidarity and self-worth in working in these communities of women. This has resulted in a 'highly significant transition from wage labour to independent production. Women eagerly speak

of the control over their time and labour that they now enjoy'
(Mukherjee-Reed 2011).

This is but one of many developments in Kerala focused on local
community autonomy, in this case on local women's communities.
It is built on a recognition that such collective action can build
social solidarity and self- and community esteem. It is not known
what the impact of this project has been on the women's health,
but all the indicators and all the evidence on social determinants of
health from elsewhere suggest that this has to be health-enhancing!

Erattupettah: the healthy village

This is the story of the remarkable efforts of Erattupettah's villagers,
very often on a voluntary basis, to make their community
healthy. These efforts occurred against a background of a recently
conducted review of health problems. This revealed various sanitation problems, with 20 per cent of the houses not having latrines,
and sewage from hotels being dumped in the river. There were
various problems with drinking water and over 400 houses were
not habitable. The Primary Health Centre was dilapidated and
poorly equipped.

In the wake of the People's Campaign the people of Erattupettah,
who previously had tried to do something about their problems but
lacked adequate resources, recognised that here was an opportunity
to make a difference. They decided to pursue the idea of a 'Healthy
Village'.

The results were far-reaching. In schools, 6,000 students were
given health check-ups. The hotels in the area that had been
dumping their sewage in the local river were compelled to construct
sewage pits, and given a sanitation certificate when they complied.
Without that certificate they could not get their licences renewed.
Of the hundreds of houses that had lacked safe latrines, 80 per cent
were equipped within four years. Safe drinking water was made
available to 1,750 families who previously could not access such
water. Solid waste management was improved. And the formerly
dilapidated Primary Health Centre, refurbished and re-equipped,
began to receive regular medical supplies. Attendances increased
from 68 per day in 1996 to 250 per day in 2000 (Elamon *et al.* 2004).

There were other improvements to facilities, all aimed at bettering the health of the local population but, importantly, doing so according to the preferences and priorities of the local community, which now had the power and the money to make these changes. Although the change in health has not been measured formally, 'Erattupettah remained free from outbreaks of cholera, acute diarrhoeal diseases, rat fever and infectious hepatitis, all of which hit neighbouring villages ... in 2001 and 2002' (Elamon *et al.* 2004).

This 'Healthy Village' is an example of how a community, when given the opportunity and the resources to make a difference to their health, can get together collectively and genuinely improve things. Whether this initiative can be sustained is a concern. We must wait and see.

Palliative care

Suchitra (2009) reports on a palliative care model that has spread throughout Kerala. It currently boasts 150 palliative clinics supported by 10,000 active trained volunteers, 85 doctors and 270 nurses looking after 25,000 patients. The coverage of palliative care patients across Kerala is 20 per cent, in comparison to a national average of 1–2 per cent. In some districts, such as Wayanad, coverage is around 70 per cent.

This all started because of one man, K. M. Basheer, a farmer who was probably 'the first non-medical person in the world to head a pain and palliative care unit' (Suchitra 2009). In 1998 a palliative society was formed at Nilambur in Malappuram District. Basheer recognised that so many chronically ill people and their families, often very poor, were struggling without social, financial or emotional support. With friends, he sought support from as many locals as possible to provide some sort of care for these people. Within the first year, 60 volunteers had been trained.

The movement spread to adjoining districts, with thousands of people volunteering to help, usually for just two hours a week. Funding is seemingly no problem, with most funds coming in small donations from the people in local communities. 'Tens of thousands of ordinary people – labourers, headload workers, autorickshaw drivers, government employees, teachers, even schoolchildren – make a small donation to keep the movement going' (Suchitra 2009).

In the wake of this in 2008 'the Kerala government – in a first for any government in Asia – came out with a palliative care policy'. It is community-based and 'considers home-based care the cornerstone of palliative care services'. It has been suggested that the model might not work elsewhere, at least not as it stands, because 'Kerala has achieved total literacy and has a high level of social and political consciousness ... but such community-based efforts could be taken as examples and new models developed for other places' (Suchitra 2009).

We should note that the source and reason for the success in developing this programme is placed yet again on literacy, together with social and political consciousness. That raises the important question of how these attributes of a society can be emulated elsewhere. I return to this issue in the Conclusion.

Coca-Cola and Kerala

Another side to Kerala is the participation and community orientation expressed in its political activism. The state has stood up to the corporation Coca-Cola and accused it of drying up local water sources and polluting the area surrounding its plant at Plachimada in Palakkad District. Indeed, in the wake of a long community campaign, in February 2011 the Kerala government passed a bill to establish a tribunal to 'realise compensation from Coca-Cola for the "environmental loss and other damages" caused by its bottling plant' (*The India Daily*, 25 February 2011). Coca-Cola responded by saying that: 'The bill is devoid of any facts or scientific data.'

This began in 2000.

> Within a year after the plant opened, local water sources started to dry up, putting hundreds of farm families out of business. All 260 bore wells installed by public authorities have gone dry. As well, the soil, water and air around the plant have become contaminated from the sludge by-product, which includes cadmium and other trace metals. What is left of the water is not fit for bathing or cooking, so high are the chlorides from waste water pumping from the plant. (Barlow, quoted in Council of Canadians 2011)

The landmark decision of February 2011 by the Kerala government to demand compensation from Coca-Cola comes after a lengthy struggle by local women. They staged daily sit-ins in front of the plant over a four-year period starting in 2002. In 2003 the water was tested by the British Broadcasting Corporation and found to contain carcinogens (cadmium and lead). The Kerala Pollution Control Board then did similar tests but with different results, suggesting the levels of carcinogens were not dangerous (but they banned the use of the biosolids as fertiliser, which was the cause of the problem, and the official who cleared the carcinogen levels was investigated for corruption) (Modus Operandi 2007).

There followed a string of legal battles between the company and the *panchayat*, with the *panchayat* ordering the plant be closed and the High Court ordering it to be reopened when Coca-Cola appealed. Effectively, however, the plant has been closed since 2004.

Modus Operandi (2007) report: 'In many ways Plachimada can be seen as a precursor of things to come, as the lowest level of society reacts to a vital resource being taken away from it for the benefit of industrial development.'

That seems a fitting conclusion on the broader front. In the context of this chapter the key point I would make is that this happened in Kerala. It might well have happened elsewhere, but this chapter has shown how Kerala has developed a strong sense of community and social solidarity, in particular a strong sense of empowerment among Keralan women but also a strong response at state level in support of local community initiatives. With the latest action at state level in passing the bill to gain compensation from Coca-Cola, that combination appears to be winning the day against the forces of this corporation. That might happen elsewhere but would be surprising. The fact that it can happen in Kerala is not unexpected.

But on this issue of the local community versus Coca-Cola, let the last word be with Veerendrakunar, a former federal minister. In a speech to the Indian parliament he stated: 'The cruel fact is that water from our underground sources is pumped out free and sold ... to make millions every day, at the same time destroying our environment and damaging the health of our people. For us rivers, dams and water sources are the property of the nation and her people' (Cockburn 2005).

In Kerala, when local community forces meet neoliberalism, the former win – or at least can win. Elsewhere?

Conclusion

I have tried in this chapter to present a flavour of Kerala and its strengths at a local community level. So often it seems the story of Kerala is told as a Keralan story and that is fine. What is important is to recognise that the true story of Kerala is at the local community level. That does not stop it being Keralan but it manifests itself in so many different ways in different local communities: with the volunteerism and the giving of small donations locally to provide palliative care for local people; by battling against a corporate giant; by believing in the power of community to build one's own "Healthy Village" according to how local people want to build it; and by women feeling empowered by a sense of community to grow food for themselves and their families and thereby build solidarity, self-respect and community respect. But it is Keralan at a state level, in that there there is a willingness to trust, believe in and support local communities, provide funding and step back. That is a real strength of Kerala. Fortunately, this stepping back is something that can be replicated elsewhere – but only if there is the political will to do so, and that means a willingness to serve the community or the communities rather than the market and the corporations, an issue I return to in the Conclusion.

16 / Cuban health care and social determinants of health: just too good for the US?

While there are changes afoot in Cuba, the way in which that country has been able to maintain high levels of population health and low inequalities has provided some important lessons for other countries over many years. It is remarkable that while Cuba's success in achieving such high health standards for a relatively low-income country are comparatively well known, the reasons why it has been so successful are so little analysed or understood. That neglect has been overcome to some extent at least in recent years, in work that I draw upon in this chapter. The neglect and the explanation for it, however, are major parts of this chapter in their own right. The lengths that the US will go to *not* to learn about and from Cuba, but to try to prevent others from learning about and from Cuba, are quite extraordinary. And why? It seems that they are so convinced of the merits of their neoliberal ways in health care and in their economy more generally that they cannot countenance any other way, especially if it is communist and right on their doorstep. (For a brief but useful account of the US embargo and blockade of Cuba see Sierra, no date.) I also want to make mention in this chapter of the neglect by conventional health economists of what Bob Evans (2008) – one of the few health economists to examine Cuban health and health care – has called 'the Cuban paradox' in a delightfully titled article to which I will return later, 'Thomas McKeown, meet Fidel Castro: physicians, population health and the Cuban paradox'.

Cuban health and health care

Spiegel and Yassi argue that 'Cuba's experience presents nothing less than a fundamental paradox or challenge to the assumption that generating wealth is the fundamental precondition for improving health – which may explain the wish by some to ignore, contest, or even hide this country's achievements' (2004: 85). This echoes the ideas of Sen that, in addition to economic growth as a road to better population health, there is the idea of support-led process which 'works through a programme of skilful social support of health care, education, and other relevant social arrangements' (2001: 338). Sen quotes the examples of 'Sri Lanka, pre-reform China, Costa Rica, or the Indian state of Kerala, which have had very rapid reductions in mortality rates and enhancement of living conditions, without much economic growth', but strangely omits Cuba from his list.

It is also the case that Cuba has not only a disease level like richer countries but a disease pattern that is more like that of a richer country, reflected in the comment from Macintyre and Hadad (2002) that Cubans 'live like the poor and die like the rich'.

Spiegel and Yassi (2004) counsel against a too-simplistic interpretation of the relationship between inequality and health, arguing that social context matters. They endorse the view of Evans and Stoddart (2003) that 'American society is characterized by a hierarchical structure defined by wealth, in which individuals experience their differences in position intensely. They [Evans and Stoddart] surmise that the correlation between economic inequality and mortality does not hold true for Canada where there are many more public services and regulatory provisions … that serve to buffer individuals against the vulnerabilities often associated with low incomes' (Spiegel and Yassi 2004: 93).

These authors and others show that Cuban health is quite remarkably good for a poor country and they attribute this to its strong emphasis on equity-orientated policies. Within health care what is most noteworthy is that Cuba has the highest ratio of doctors to population anywhere in the world (indeed, additionally it provides thousands of doctors to several developing countries each year).

It must be emphasised, however, that it is not just the health-care system that is contributing to the good health of Cubans. Education is excellent and compulsory up to the twelfth grade. Adult literacy is nearly 97 per cent. The testing of students in third and fourth grade shows Cuba at the top in comparison to the other Latin American countries. Much, indeed most, housing is public. Individuals are permitted to buy and sell their homes but at prices set by government. Employment was close to being full up until the 'Special Period' in the early 1990s, which was the time following the withdrawal of Soviet support. This has been problematical since. Officially unemployment runs at less than 2 per cent but this figure excludes those in the informal sector. Recently there have been moves to shift more than one million people out of state employment who have been underemployed working for the state. They are being re-employed in construction and agriculture, joining cooperatives, or becoming self-employed.

All of this is despite an embargo/blockade imposed by the US on travel and goods since 1960, which continues to this day. It has been of varying severity and coverage, but for most of the time and still today covers medicines and health-care supplies. At times, too, it has banned US aid to any country which trades with Cuba (Sierra, no date).

Yet despite the withdrawal of Soviet support and at the same time an intensification of the US blockade, including of medicine and other health-related supplies, as Spiegel and Yassi show, 'the trend toward improvement [in population health] persisted over the course of the decade' of the 1990s (2004: 88).

Bob Evans (2008) has sought to try to explain this Cuban phenomenon. He latches on to the very high doctor-to-population ratio of nearly 6:1000, the highest in the world as noted above. But investigating the idea that in an international context lots of doctors leads to good population health, he cannot get much traction on that hypothesis.

What Evans then does is to argue what Sen (2001) suggests (as above) across populations, namely that it is not necessarily the quantity of resources (for Evans doctors, for Sen GDP) that matters in improving health, but what you do with them. Thus Evans contends that the

> difference appears to be that in Cuba, primary care physician (and nurse) teams have responsibility for the health of geographically defined populations, not merely of those patients who come in the door. These teams are then linked to community- and higher-level

political organisations that both hold them accountable for the health of their populations and provide them with channels through which to influence the relevant non-medical determinants. To take on these roles, the *medico familiar integrale* (MFI) is trained in both the medical and the non-medical aspects of health. (2008: 31)

Here we have a combination of a number of things, but most importantly we have a local community focus, a marriage of health-care and non-health-care health-promoting considerations (all as social determinants of health) and last, but perhaps the most vital ingredient of all, political power and accountability both to influence the non-medical variables and to shift power to where it needs to be – with the citizens.

The WHO Commission on Social Determinants of Health (WHO 2008) did give considerable prominence to Cuban success. For example, a background paper prepared for the Commission states: 'Post-revolutionary Cuba constitute[s] an important example of "good health at low cost" … Cuba's population health profile more closely resembles wealthy countries' (Irwin and Scali 2005). The authors then consider some of the reasons for this:

The principles of universality, equitable access and governmental control guided post-revolutionary Cuban health policies, which focused on achieving social equity through free provision of needed services, including medical care, diagnostic tests and vaccines for 13 preventable diseases. Cuba's public health policy prioritises health promotion and disease prevention activities, decentralisation, intersectoral action and community participation; it features a local primary care approach which exists within an organised system of consultation and referral for more specialised care. At local level, physicians and nurses live within the community they serve and provide not only clinical diagnosis and treatment, but also community education about general health issues and non-medical health determinants.

Thus Cuba represents a society which has chosen the egalitarian and 'cheap' route to good health. It has embraced key features of the social determinants of health and shown that success in terms of good population health indicators can be achieved in practical ways. The egalitarianism of Cuba, the active participation of the community in health planning, and the potential impact of the social determinants of health more generally are all features that are highly relevant to what I am proposing as a better way forward for health and health care more generally. What is remarkable about Cuba's success is just how little Cuba's health and health care have been analysed by 'mainstream' health economists. Yet as Aviva Chomsky notes, the commitment to health is notable. 'First, the government understands health to be the responsibility of the state. Second, the government approaches health as a social issue that includes health-care delivery but is far from limited to it' (2000: 333).

Cuban health and the US

Above and beyond the fact that being a communist state makes Cuba a perceived threat to the US, the nature and causes of its success with respect to health are also threatening to the medical and health-care establishments of the US. The market in the US, despite the enormous costs of health care, the relatively poor standards of health of the US population, and the gross inequities of that system, remains king. As I indicated in Chapter 5, the fact that Obama's health-care reforms can be dubbed socialist seems quite extraordinary. When they are set along side the almost pathological loathing in the United States of all things Cuban, however, and the various attempts to use military and economic means to destroy the regime and to try to stop the spread of knowledge of the Cuban success story with respect to health, Obama being called a socialist makes more sense.

Ochoa and Lopez Pardo (1997) have shown that Cuba, by introducing rationing for essential food items at subsidised rates, was able to improve nutritional standards. The arts and sports are areas where Cuba has also excelled internationally. One remarkable aspect of Cuba's success is that a US State Department-sponsored study was set up specifically to cast doubt on Cuba's success in health! One can only marvel at the lengths to which the US will go to try to bring down the Cuban regime and to discredit its successes simply because it is a communist regime. What is particularly interesting about this study is that, according to Spiegel and Yassi (2004: 89), this backfired and 'only served to acknowledge Cuba's achievements'.

Perhaps this irrational US fear of Cuba's success in delivering a healthy population from very low resources is fed by the narrow gap in the health status of the two populations and the significant difference in costs. Indeed the most recent life expectancy figures suggest they are neck and neck on 78.3 years, while the difference in annual expenditure per capita in current US dollars is astonishing: Cuba $707 and the US $7410 (World Bank 2011). Given this situation, it is remarkable to discover – as I did in researching for this chapter – how little is published on Cuban health and health care. As Cooper *et al.* write:

> After the revolution of 1959 ... Cuba acquired the pariah status of a wayward child and has been variously vilified in rhetoric, attacked militarily and economically, and consigned to cultural oblivion.... Despite occasional 'discovery pieces' the biomedical literature in English has been almost entirely silent on the Cuban experience and US government policy temporarily forbade publication of articles from Cuba by US journals or their foreign subsidiaries. (2006: 817)

This censorship by the US of publications on Cuba is perhaps the strongest (but surely most bizarre) symptom of US paranoia with respect to Cuba.

True to this sentiment, what little does manage to get published is so often vilified. For example Drain and Barry (2010) presented the following argument in support of Cuban health care:

> Despite the blockade, Cuba has achieved better healthcare results than most Latin American countries and comparable with those of most of the developed nations. Cuba's average life expectancy is the highest (78.6 years) and it also has the highest density of medical doctors per capita – 59 doctors to 10,000 people – and the lowest mortality rate for children under one year of age (5.0 per 1,000 live births) and infant mortality (7.0 per 1,000 live births) among the 33 countries of Latin America and the Caribbean.... In 2006, the Cuban government allocated about $355 per capita for healthcare.... The annual healthcare cost assigned to an American citizen that same year was $6,714.

They were then attacked on the basis that theirs was an 'egregious misrepresentation of the Cuban health-care system' (Hirschfeld 2010) and asked by Bodenstein (2010) 'to speculate on what the quality of health care in Cuba would be were it only based on discoveries and medical advances originating in Cuba'!

In 2009, President Barack Obama extended the US embargo against Cuba. At that time, Amnesty International Secretary-General Irene Khan appealed for its lifting, stating that it was preventing Cubans from benefiting from vital medicines and medical equipment essential for their health (Amnesty International 2009).

In January 2011, Obama did introduce some slight easing of the embargo by allowing Cuban Americans to travel to Cuba and telecom company investment in Cuba. The easing of the embargo also meant that students, academic staff and religious groups would be free to visit Cuba (MacCaskill 2011). Further, Americans will be allowed to send up to $500 to support private economic and other activities, though not any involving the Cuban Communist Party or its members. There is no relaxation on medical or health-care supplies.

Not that all US citizens or US doctors agree with the embargo. In a 'Statement from the American Public Health Association' Diane Kuntz (1996) writes:

> Public health professionals who have served in other countries have long held up the Cuban health-care system as a model. In Cuba all citizens have a right to high-quality health care, to education, to day care, and to other social services. The infant mortality rate, life expectancy, and other health indicators in Cuba match those in the world's richest countries.... It is often said that Cuba is no longer a threat to the US. But that's not true. It is a threat. The threat lies in the example Cuba offers – an example of a country with the political will to provide good health care to all its citizens.... The US is fighting this threat – using food, medicine, and medical supplies as weapons. In part as a result of the embargo, many essential products are in short supply in Cuba. Soap, laboratory equipment, textbooks – all kinds of basic goods are scarce. Cuban doctors must count every pill and measure every drop of medicine they dispense. Cuban citizens – especially children and elderly people – are suffering the consequences of our government's policy.

And the writer calls for an end to the embargo.

Also, in 2004, the Minnesota Medical Association put the following motion to the American Medical Association (Minnesota Medical Association 2004): 'That the Minnesota Medical

Association support[s] the institution of humanitarian aid to Cuba immediately to prevent further disease and death on the island' and they submitted 'a resolution ... requesting that the AMA lobby Congress to support efforts to remove the blockade against Cuba for humanitarian aid and to institute humanitarian aid to the country of Cuba'. I can find no record of what happened to it. Not unexpectedly it seems to have sunk without trace.

Conclusion

Writing in *Frontline*, the national magazine of India, Sivaraman (1998) summed up the difference between the US and Cuba as follows:

> The UN has declared poverty – defined not just as poverty of income but as poverty from a 'human development perspective i.e. a denial of choices and opportunities for living a tolerable life' – as a denial of human rights. Applying this criterion, the US is more of a human rights offender – with 15 per cent of its population under poverty against Cuba's 5 per cent. What is probably crucial for making life tolerable is whether the polity is governed by the morality of the market or is of a humane kind.

Sivaraman (*ibid.*) then quotes Noam Chomsky:

> Outrage [in the US] peaked during the Pan-American games held in the United States, when Cuban athletes failed to succumb to a huge propaganda campaign to induce them to defect, including lavish financial offers to become professional; they felt a commitment to their country and its people, they told reporters.

The extent of denialism evoked by the success of Cuba in delivering health is startling. It is ideological. It is an unwillingness bordering on pathological to argue that the market is always right and always better and that there cannot be exceptions. Yet Cuba so clearly is succeeding not only at home but in what it does beyond its shores in exporting thousands of doctors to so many poor countries across the globe – and this despite the embargo of Cuba by the US, now over 50 years old.

The impact of the embargo is major and continuous. Just as I was finalising the text of this book, I came across this report for the

Cuban government dated June 2011. 'In January, the government of the United States of America saw fit to seize $4.207 million in funds allocated to Cuba by the UN Global Fund to Fight AIDS, Tuberculosis and Malaria for the first quarter of 2011' (Blum 2011).

Cuba, however, does manage to provoke some 'positive retaliation' from the US – in the shape of the US Naval Ship *Comfort*. This has '12 operating rooms and a 1,000–bed hospital' and provides 'hundreds of thousands of free surgeries in places such as Belize, Guatemala, Panama, El Salvador, Peru, Ecuador, Colombia, Nicaragua and Haiti'. Sadly, this venture has been described by Peter Hakim, president of the Inter-American Dialogue, a pro-US policy-research group in Washington, in the following terms: 'It makes us look like we're trying to imitate them. Cuba's doctors aren't docked at port for a couple of days, but are in the country for years'.

If more US citizens knew more of Cuba, many would want the US to do more 'imitation' closer to home. But then perhaps Obama would need to be a real socialist!

17 / Venezuela: power to the community

The recent shifts in power and in institutions in Venezuela focus very much on the community rather than individuals as decision-making entities. These follow the coming to power of Hugo Chavez in 1999. This case study will be analysed not only to evaluate how successful it has been but also to examine how transferable it might be to other countries.

The Venezuelan model is described by Muntaner *et al.* (2007). It emphasises primary care, based on community participation in decision making and funded by the public sector. 'This integrated model of care emphasises a holistic approach to health and illness through the coordination of [the primary health care organisation with others] addressing education, food security, public sanitation and employment, among other key social determinants of health' (*ibid.*: 317). These authors show that 'people lacking potable water who suffer from recurring intestinal infections are not only prescribed the appropriate antibiotics but also encouraged to organise to demand adequate access to clean water' (*ibid.*). The organisational structure is such that 'health teams and patients are supported by Health Committees comprised of [community] residents'. It is in this way that the local community residents 'exercise their participation in primary health care clinics' (*ibid.*).

There is no reason, say Muntaner *et al.*, why this model could not be used in the West (*ibid.*: 319). This is not a textbook example of a health policy built on the paradigm of this book, but it is an approximate case study of one system that adheres to a number of the facets of the paradigm. I believe we can all learn much from a closer examination of Venezuelan health and health care.

The revolution in Venezuelan health care

It is worth noting that while Venezuela has been a democracy since 1958, access to health care for much of that time was far from democratic. While theoretically all had access to free care, the reality was that such access depended on where you were in the society and what connections you had. In the 1980s and 1990s most growth in health spending was in the private sector, with inevitable consequences for equity in health and health care. While the public health-care spend had been 13.3 per cent of the total public expenditure in 1970, this fell to 9.3 per cent in 1990 and to 7.9 per cent in 1996. That 1996 figure was equivalent to just 1.73 per cent of national income (PAHO 2006). Conditions were no better with respect to key social determinants of health. In 1990 nearly a third of homes were without piped water. In 1996, 42.5 per cent of the population were officially deemed to be living in extreme poverty (PAHO 2006).

This is how PAHO summed it up:

> During the 1990s, the response capacity of the health-care network was officially insufficient. There were long waiting lists for surgery and specialised outpatient care, and often there were not enough essential supplies to provide the care needed. The network did not have plans for preparing for or mitigating emergencies and disasters. This situation, created by public underfunding, led to the decision to privatise the health services and relieve the State of full responsibility for guaranteeing the right to health.

It is important to recognise that this is where the Venezuelan health services were *before* reforms occurred. Had the movement to bring about radical change not happened, it seems clear that Venezuelan health care would have continued to be grossly underfunded, with a very real prospect that the great majority of what spending there was would have been in the private sector. The reforms did not happen in a vacuum, nor did they come from a vacuum.

The Venezuelan Constitution of 1999 guarantees everyone the right to free health care. This is done through a public, government-funded system based on what is called Mision Barrio Adentro, which means 'Mission inside the neighbourhood'. In the 1980s and 1990s the Venezuelan economy struggled and public services were cut, including public health services. Initial efforts in the early 2000s to deliver better health services to the poor failed. However, by 2004 this form of care, Mision Barrio Adentro, was spreading across the country. It was a movement based in the communities and was extended nationally when an agreement was reached between Venezuela and Cuba to provide Cuban doctors to staff the programme, while Venezuela provided Cuba with much needed oil and medicines. The process of reform is driven by local communities and also relies on close ties between these communities and the doctors who undertake to live in the communities. The doctors share the same lifestyle as the community. These doctors are well suited for this situation as they are trained in Cuba in what is called 'general integrated medicine' which is 'a specialty emphasising familial, community, and environmental contexts and a critical approach to the intersection between biological, epidemiological, social and humanitarian dimensions' (Briggs and Mantini-Briggs 2009). It is a democratisation of health care as Chavez (2009) has called it. Participation in decision making at a local community level is an integral part of the whole system.

While Chavez did not 'invent' this new form of delivery of health care to the poor, he saw its merits and provided much-needed resources to help it to spread throughout Venezuela. The 'equality' between the community and in turn the patient and the doctor is a key to the success of the system. It is not driven by the state but in reality is facilitated by the state. It is not controlled by the medical profession; the doctors play a crucial role in the system but they are very much a part of it rather than seeking an agency role in how the system is to operate. In other words there is a very real shift in power to the people in the Venezuelan health-care system.

It is also the case – which is an enormous bonus – that the doctors involved are trained not just in medicine but in health more generally, and are thus well placed to pursue and advocate for the social determinants of health in the communities in which they work (see Evans 2008 for the same observation in the case of Cuba). The involvement of Cuba and its doctors followed in the wake of a refusal by Venezuelan doctors to take part in this new scheme. Indeed, the doctors went on strike to oppose the scheme.

McNulty (2009) sums up the movement towards health care for all:

> popular participation, preventative medicine, and evaluation of community health issues ... Barrio Adentro began constructing clinics within neighborhoods where many had never been to a doctor. Through this program, a community can organise to receive funding to build a clinic and bring in doctors. The community is responsible for creating health committees, the members of which go door to door to assess the specific health issues of their community. Doctors who live in the communities also make house calls. People participate in the process of serving the health needs of the entire population.

Starting with prevention, the programme has harnessed the power (and the real needs) of communities across a wide spectrum. McNulty describes how it

> has expanded to include emergency health services, mental health services, surgeries, cancer treatment, dental care, access to optometrists as well as free glasses and contact lenses, support systems for those with disabilities and their families, as well as access to a large variety of medical specialists.... Instead of a for-profit industry systematically denying access to large sectors of the population, health care in Venezuela is seen as a basic human right. No one is turned away, and no one is denied care. In Venezuela, they treat [the] whole person, not simply their illness. (McNulty 2009)

Does it work?

There are a variety of indicators to show that the system works. For example Westhoff *et al.* (2010) show figures for before and after 18 months of the implementation of the Barrio Adentro. The number of primary care doctors rose from 1,500 to 13,000. Consultations with patients went up from 3.5 million to 17 million; primary care centres from 4,400 (but only 1,500 with a doctor) to 5,500, all with doctors. The health effects? 'It is estimated that 16,400 lives were saved, over 800 births were attended, 161,800 vaccinations were given, 13 million prescription medications were dispensed, and 22 million health education activities were provided.'

Additionally, the same authors suggest there were some positive 'side effects', although I think many of these are better seen in terms of the social determinants of health. These 'created new employment opportunities, provided education and training for those who are interested in health and medicine as careers, strengthened the cooperation and capacity within communities, consolidated the first line of health care, and have given dignity and rights to those who were previously underserved' (*ibid.*). There was also a 30 per cent reduction in presentations at emergency departments in Caracas alone.

Transferable elsewhere?

There seems no reason in principle why this Barrio Adentro system cannot be replicated elsewhere with suitable modifications for local cultural and resource considerations. What is needed, though, are several things. First, a recognition that the way an existing system is currently operating is in some sense wrong. That can be at a number of levels – inefficiently, inequitably, in moral terms, or, more generally, not in the interests of the broad population. Second, this kind of shift concerns who holds power, both in the society and in the health-care system. That issue, so seldom addressed with respect to health-care systems, has to be recognised as being potentially problematical. When there are neoliberal governments in power, these will tend to see health care as being something that they want to be treated as a commodity for those who can afford to see it in these terms. For the poor and disadvantaged, such governments will want to adopt a paternalistic approach and, together with the medical profession in the form of the national medical association, determine what sort of health care and what sort of health-care system people are to get. Getting power to the people is crucial; overcoming the lack of understanding of the necessity of this is perhaps the biggest hurdle of all. It is a hurdle that the medical profession wants to preserve because that is the main source of their power. They will not lightly part with it, and Venezuela was fortunate to be able to get round that difficulty by importing Cuban doctors. But the necessity of addressing these issues has to come from governments who are prepared to place health above the power and profits of vested interests, and give that power over to the people at a community level.

There is much literature on what is called the 'agency relationship' in health care (see, for example, Vick and Scott 1998), which is where the individual doctor helps the individual patient to decide what is good for him or her (the patient). The balance here is inevitably tricky and will vary between different doctors and different patients, and even one patient in different situations. Such questions arise as: whose 'best' is being assessed in deciding what the best course of action is? Who is doing the assessment? Best in terms of the patient's health or well-being, or what? It is understandable that this agency relationship has spawned much literature and attention from doctors, consumer groups, health policy makers, economists, ethicists and so on – it is an important issue.

What is the 'agency relationship' around health-care systems? I cannot think that this expression has been used in that context and yet the shift in Venezuela is perhaps best seen in just this way. It is about who is to decide what sort of health-care system Venezuelans are to have. Is it to be determined top-down by politicians, senior policy makers and experts? Or bottom-up – where 'the bottom' is the doctors and their representatives? Or the consumers or patient representatives who sit on various committees but are in fact powerless? Or is it the community?

If we look again at the South African system as an example of not going down the Venezuelan road, the parallels of South Africa today with Venezuela in the 1980s and 1990s are very great. South Africa has a strongly neoliberal government and a public health-care system that is grossly underfunded, alongside a higher-quality, expensive private system. It has a very unequal society, with the great majority living in poverty. What road will South Africa take? Certainly there are efforts being made currently to bring in a National Health Insurance scheme, although that is being vehemently opposed by the private sector (see Chapter 7). That sector agrees on the need to improve the public sector, but wants the private sector left alone.

This is about power. In South Africa what is fascinating is that the voice of the people is not there at the negotiating table over National Health Insurance. The 'experts' and the private sector are present in force, but there has been all too little attempt to try to find out what the people want. That lack is reflected in the Green

Paper on the NHI published in August 2011 (Department of Health 2011). Yet the Barrio Adentro would be so apposite for South Africa! Crucial in such a move would be obtaining appropriately trained doctors, and perhaps again Cuba could help – but to go down this road there would need to be, early, a major shift in the training of South African doctors.

PAHO reports: 'Ratification of the new Constitution [for Venezuela] in 1999 sparked the collective construction of a new economic and social model' which is 'guided by the affirmation that health is a fundamental social right guaranteed by the Venezuelan state, based on co-responsibility on the part of all citizens and guaranteed active participation by organised communities' (2006: 21).

Interestingly the South African constitution states: 'Everyone has the right to have access to

• health care services, including reproductive health care;
• sufficient food and water; and social security, including, if they are unable to support themselves and their dependants, appropriate social assistance.'

Further, 'The state must take reasonable legislative and other measures, within its available resources, to achieve the progressive realisation of each of these rights.'

The wording of the two constitutions – the Venezuelan and the South African – is not so very different. The sentiments seem very similar. Yet the outcomes in health and health care are immensely different. Why? First, Venezuela has abandoned the neoliberal road while South Africa is yet more wedded to it. Second, the Venezuelan constitution makes direct reference to a principle 'based on co-responsibility on the part of all citizens and guaranteed active participation by organised communities'. Its South African counterpart has not gone down this community empowerment route.

Conclusion

The Venezuelan model is the closest that I can find to a working example of what my paradigm would point towards. The emphasis is on the community, community values and community power; the shift away from a neoliberal state; the disempowering of the medical profession; and the role of the state being restricted to financing and facilitating.

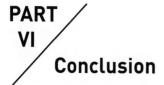

PART VI

Conclusion

Conclusion: can we change?

What I have sought to do in this book is to expose, primarily by way of examples, why as a planet we are failing to get to grips with providing health to the global population. This is despite having such abundant resources, quite amazing technology, remarkably skilled health-care personnel and wonder drugs. It is also despite seemingly well-intended endeavours over the MDGs, support for HIV/AIDS victims and the generosity of the people of the globe when tsunamis, earthquakes or other disasters befall.

In some situations health is getting a little better and I do not want the arguments of this book to be dismissed by defenders of the status quo because I have not acknowledged that. The statistics, however, are at best mixed.

Why do we fail?

But what is the goal here? Is it simply to do a little bit better and in just some situations? Surely not. We can do much better than we are doing, especially for the poor generally, but most particularly for those trying to survive on less than $2 a day. I quoted Thomas Pogge (2008) in the Introduction: 'Many more people – some 360 million – have died from hunger and remediable diseases in peacetime in the 20 years since the end of the Cold War than have perished from wars, civil wars, and government repression over the entire twentieth century.'

Pogge (2008) also has this to say on the issue of poverty, which is so closely associated with poor health:

Citizens of the rich countries are ... conditioned to downplay the severity and persistence of world poverty and to think of it as an occasion for minor charitable assistance. This widespread lack of attention to the world poverty problem becomes morally indefensible once we understand that its human cost is enormous, that its economic magnitude is pathetically small by comparison, and that it has barely diminished during recent periods of healthy global economic growth.

Why do we fail so miserably and grasp at straws of minor success? What I have tried to show is that the problem lies in the global political economy. Indeed, as I write this (August 2011) the IMF has just appointed a French woman, Ms Christine Lagarde, as its new chief. She is European, which is the key qualification for the post, just as being from the US is the key qualification for heading up the World Bank. Lagarde was elected 'by consensus' by the governing board of the IMF.

Democracy? No. The South African Finance Minister, Pravin Gordhan, has recently argued (*The New Age* 2011) that the IMF should move towards a democratic system to choose the institution's next leader.

We are talking about a shift from a decades-old tradition to a new way of doing things. We're talking about a shift from an entitlement to heading certain institutions to a more democratic process.... This is an important institution and I think there are also important historical issues at stake, whether the institution continue to operate in the old way, whether the twenty-first century has indeed arrived for everyone concerned.

His plea and that of other developing nations fell on deaf ears.

By and large we know what to do to improve health. We have on the planet the resources to do it. Yet we don't act. Those who have the power to bring about that improvement do not care.

Wars are waged and justified trying to make a better world. The US has spent $429 billion in Afghanistan chasing bin Laden. He was eventually killed but not in Afghanistan. His death seems not to have made any difference to the geopolitical terrorist scene.

Afghanistan has a population of 30 million. That money could have provided humanitarian aid to the Afghan people amounting to over $14,000 to each Afghan or over $1,400 to each in each of these 10 years. The GDP per capita of that country in 2008, the last year for which figures are available, was $800.

The rich countries of the West steal doctors and nurses from the poor. The rich provide themselves with good (private) health care. That protects their health and also their wallets – as otherwise, through taxes, they would have to pay for the care of the poor.

The rich countries of the West sign on with the UN to deliver 0.7 per cent of their national incomes to provide aid to poor countries – that is not a lot – but then most fail to get near to 0.7 per cent. Out of all the OECD countries the US – and Greece – are at the bottom, not managing even a quarter of that 0.7 per cent. At the same time deregulated financial systems transfer more funds from South to North than aid flows from North to South (Weston 2011).

The pharmaceutical companies focus on those who can pay and by and large ignore the poor because they are not good consumers from a profit-making perspective. These companies are supported in their endeavours by the so-called 'world trade' organisation, the WTO. This covers a large part of the world but is not run by the 'world' but by a few Western governments, and certainly not by any group that might fit the description of the global community. It is not about world trade but about protecting the profits of the transnational corporations. The undemocratic World Bank and the equally undemocratic IMF impose their neoliberal punitive policies – euphemistically called 'structural adjustment programmes' – on the poor in the interests of global profit making.

The World Health Organization is seen in some quarters as increasingly under the influence of corporations. The People's Health Movement (2011) has drawn attention to the illegitimate power of these corporates by ridiculing 'the WHO's unprecedented invitation to Microsoft CEO Bill Gates to address the inaugural session of the 58th World Health Assembly as one of its keynote speakers' which it sees 'as an inappropriate development which they fear could signal an increase in undue corporate influence on ... WHO'. The PHM is demanding that 'Microsoft Corporation be declared an honorary "member country" of the World Health Organisation'!

This book has been highly critical of the structurally unjust (and uncaring) world we live in and its failure across the planet and in the vast majority of countries to address the global burden of disease. The inequities have been exposed as worsening not only between the rich nations of the North and the nations of the South but between the rich and poor within nations. Strictly this is not a North–South issue. It is a rich–poor issue. Yet more fundamentally, it is a power issue which is based in class.

That issue of class power needs to be addressed and redressed. It has been exacerbated over the last three decades with the advent of neoliberalism. That has done little if anything to help the poor; it has created yet greater social divisions and inequalities. Governments, including those which are supposedly democratic, work in collusion with corporations.

Health-care systems have ceased to be social institutions, as health care has been seen more and more as a commodity and attempts to reform it – at least in the US – as 'socialist'. The UK National Health Service is threatened by market forces. Low- and middle-income countries, where inevitably the poor struggle to make any payments for health care, are increasingly pushed in the direction of more and more private care. They are encouraged down this privatisation road by the World Bank. This is true not only of health care; they are encouraged to privatise more and more of their economies by both the World Bank and the IMF. Thus countries which fall into debt and need loans are then forced down the neoliberal road through 'structural adjustment programmes'.

Global warming – this enormous threat to global health – is denied and then largely ignored. The evidence that it is happening and happening fast is there, but is undermined by attacks from all sorts of quarters – driven mainly and directly by the neoliberal demands for economic growth and enhanced profits. The World Bank, the supposed guardian of the planet in issues around global warming, gives a massive grant to the neoliberal South African government to power ahead with heavily polluting coal-fired generating stations.

Can we change?

Yes we can change and as the book has demonstrated there are existing models that we can draw on in Cuba, Venezuela and Kerala, for example. These community-focused societies and health-care systems show not only that a different political economy of health and health care is possible. It can deliver health.

The approach suggested in this book looks at a communitarian approach to health and health care. It argues for a shift in power from the current structures to give 'power to the people' – the critically informed people. It suggests that health care is best seen as a social institution and that societies must become more genuinely democratic with much more participation in decision making, in setting principles and priorities. It argues that people care and that they seek equity in health and health care. They see health-care systems as part of the social fabric and a caring health-care system as a part of a decent society. They are too seldom asked what sort of health-care system they want; even less often are they asked what sort of society they want, as elections are increasingly between 'the centre right' and 'the centre right', the twenty-first-century equivalent of Tweedledum and Tweedledee.

To move the power base, the use of deliberative democracy techniques is essential so that critically informed people can again take more control over their lives and their institutions. Such participation is the mechanism for the power shift. The location for future power is the critically informed community.

In addition to the merits of this as a power shift, the focus on participation and community in itself is likely to be health-enhancing. It moves on from the individualism that neoliberalism has engendered in so many societies and brings empowerment and social solidarity in its wake. The caring that neoliberalism has largely destroyed can be rekindled by stressing the importance of community and participation.

The concept of community and in turn communitarianism must be extended to all levels of society and the globe. There are or can be national communities just as there can be a global one. At the global level this will mean the dismantling of the WHO, the WTO, the World Bank and the IMF and rebuilding organisations which are more genuinely reflective of world opinion and, ideally, world citizen opinion. This idea is relevant to health and health care but also more generally with respect to aid and its disbursement, how that is determined in size and nature, who pays and who receives. Perhaps most crucially, the building of a global community voice is needed as we enter the epoch of global warming. Currently nation states and their governments seem only to be interested in 'the national interest' and are incapable of looking to the planet as a whole – while corporations, driven by short-term profit-seeking, add to the narrow focus and fail to grapple with global and/or long-term strategic goals.

Creating the local community structures seems manageable; moving from there to the global is tricky. Organisations do exist that have some of the attributes we might be looking for, such as the People's Health Movement. Raffer and Singer argue for a new reciprocity between richer and poorer countries:

> There is ... a need for a new relationship between the richer and the poorer countries.... The richer countries feel like unwilling dispensers of favour imposing strict discipline as conditions for their favours ... while the poorer countries feel they do not really own the policies imposed on them but they are beggars who cannot be choosers ... the right way forward is ... by way of development contracts, genuine contracts in which both sides make clearly defined and voluntarily entered commitments, and remain in continuing consultation to adjust the contract in the light of unforeseen new circumstances. Conditionality must become a two-way business. (2001: 14)

These authors suggest that to have their proposals implemented requires an 'independent panel of arbitrators' (*ibid.*: 248). They see such a body as being 'composed of independent experts selected by the UN General Assembly.... It could dispose of funds raised by international taxation to finance measures against poverty.' That is one way to go and represents an improvement on what we have – but it is not enough. As a minimum, the citizens need to have their voices heard *directly* to be able to influence the nature of the principles to be used to underpin the social determinants of health and of health-care systems. The 'independent panel of arbitrators' might well be useful, but they should not be left to devise these principles.

Backed by the idea of the ecological debt to fund the necessary movement of resources from rich to poor, there is room for optimism. Global warming is an enormous threat not only to health but to human survival. That threat can become a promise of a better, fairer world if it can be seen in these terms and action taken quickly to avert the otherwise certain tragedy.

To date the health issues around world poverty and inequality have largely passed health economists by. The WHO commissions on Macroeconomics and Health and on Social Determinants of Health both failed to address the issue of neoliberalism and the structure of the global economy. While we have become used to the denialism surrounding global warming, denialism when it emanates from two WHO commissions is less readily recognized. It seems the influence of neoliberalism is present in these commissions. We know it was with the CME, since it was chaired by Jeffrey Sachs. As for the SDH Commission, as discussed in Chapter 4, it seems that in their deliberations the members of this Commission recognised the problems for health of neoliberalism – but when it came to making recommendations that might have addressed these problems, the Commission fell silent. We can only wonder why.

I have sought to argue that, for health-care systems and with respect to the social determinants of health, the community as the guardians of social institutions must rule. Individual communities, locally and nationally, must also have much more say in what constitute *their* social determinants of health, since these will vary from society to society. How to address them will also be something on which the community should be involved – and this is true whether that be a local community, a national community or a global community.

It is not enough simply to get citizens to reveal their preferences when evaluating health and other outcomes and processes. We need them to reveal their informed reflective preferences for what they see as the benefits (or 'the good') of health care and of public health. In other words, it is not enough to say for example what the preferences are in QALYs for quality of life versus quantity of life, with the analyst predetermining what is in the objective function. It is for the citizens to set 'the constitution' for the social institutions of health care and public health.

On the basis of my own work in Australia with citizens' juries in health care (Mooney 2010) I would make the following observations which may not hold good elsewhere but I suspect do to a considerable extent.

Critically informed citizens appear to be more compassionate and more concerned for social justice than is currently reflected in many health-care systems or societies or election results. They are much more concerned with equity. Second, staying with this equity theme allows me to address the fear that some critics have that 'ordinary citizens' simply cannot cope with such complex issues. This statement (Mooney and Blackwell 2004) is the basis of a definition of equity established by a citizens' jury in Perth in Western Australia.

> Equal access for equal need, where equality of access means that two or more groups face barriers of the same height and where the judgement of the heights is made by each group for their own group; where need is defined as capacity to benefit; and where nominally equal benefits may be weighted according to social preferences such that the benefits to more disadvantaged groups may have a higher weight attached to them than those to the better off.

I have studied equity in health care a lot in my career. I do not think I have come across a better, fuller definition than this one from a bunch of 'ignorant ordinary' citizens! The idea that critically informed citizens cannot cope with complex issues is wrong.

There is a need for a new political economy of health, where Vicente Navarro has trod a rather lonely path for too long. That needs to be very firmly about health and not just health care. It also needs to deal with health-care systems and public health as social institutions. Citizens value these institutions and not just for their outcomes.

That political economy of health must analyse the impacts of neoliberalism on health both within individual countries but also globally. It must also examine the global instruments of neoliberalism – the World Bank, the WHO, the WTO, the G8 and the IMF. Their reform is urgent. It will become more urgent with global warming. Global citizenry is absent from these bodies as are, in terms of any meaningful concept of democracy, many of the governments of the poorer countries of the world.

References

ABC *Four Corners* (2005) 'Something in the air', http://www.abc.net.au/4corners/content/2005/s1471209.htm, accessed June 2011.

Acción Ecológica (2005) 'What is ecological debt?', http://www.ecologicaldebt.org/What-is-Ecological-Debt/, accessed June 2011.

ACT Health Council (2010) 'Citizens' Jury on health priorities 2010', ACT Health Council report, http://www.health.act.gov.au/c/health?a=sendfile&ft=p&fid=1293068459&sid=, accessed June 2011.

Adams, V. (2004) 'Equity of the ineffable: cultural and political constraints in ethnomedicine as a health problem in contemporary Tibet', WP Series No. 99.05, Harvard Center for Population and Development Studies.

Amnesty International (2009) 'Obama renews Cuba trade embargo', http://www.amnesty.org/en/news-and-updates/news/obama-renews-cuba-trade-embargo-20090915, accessed June 2011.

Anderson K. and A. Bows (2011) 'Beyond "dangerous" climate change: emission scenarios for a new world', *Philosophical Transactions of the Royal Society* 369 (1934): 20–44.

Anderson, K., W. Martin and D. van der Mensgrugghe (2006) 'Global impacts of the Doha scenarios on poverty' in T. W. Hertel and L. A. Winters (eds), *Poverty and the WTO*. Washington DC: World Bank.

Angell, M. (2004) *The Truth about the Drug Companies*. New York NY: Random House.

Arrow, K. (1963) 'Uncertainty and the welfare economics of medical care', *American Economic Review* 5: 941–67.

Avineri, S. (1974) *Hegel's Theory of the Modern State*. Cambridge: Cambridge University Press.

Avineri, S. and A. de-Shalit (eds) (1992) *Communitarianism and Individualism*. Oxford: Oxford University Press.

Background Briefing ABC (2002) 'Alcoa's bad odour', http://www.abc.net.au/rn/talks/bbing/stories/s579605.htm, accessed June 2011.

Barnard, D. (2002) 'In the High Court of South Africa, Case No. 4138/98:

the global politics of access to low-cost AIDS drugs in poor countries'. *Kennedy Institute of Ethics Journal* 12 (2): 159–74.

Bevan, A. (1952) *In Place of Fear*. London: Heinemann, http://www.sochealth.co.uk/history/placeofear.htm, accessed June 2011.

Beveridge, Sir W. (1942) *Social Insurance and Allied Services*. London: HMSO.

Blum, W. (2011) 'US targeting of Cuba's health-care system', http://www.commondreams.org/view/2011/06/04-3, accessed June 2011.

Bodenstein, L. (2010) 'Cuban health care: benefits without costs', *Science* 329 (6 August): 628.

Bond, P. (2002) *Unsustainable South Africa: environment, development and social protest*. Pietermaritzburg: University of Natal Press.

—— (2005) 'Privatisation, participation and protest in the restructuring of municipal services', http://www.africanwater.org/ppp_debate1.htm, accessed June 2011.

—— (2010) 'South Africa's bubble meets boiling urban social protest', *Monthly Review* 62 (2).

Bretton Woods (1946) 'United Nations Monetary and Financial Conference at Bretton Woods. Summary of Agreements, 22 July 1944', http://www.ibiblio.org/pha/policy/1944/440722a.html, accessed 21 December 2007.

Briggs, C. L. and C. Mantini-Briggs (2009) 'Confronting health disparities: Latin American social medicine in Venezuela', *American Journal of Public Health* 99 (3): 549–55.

Broome, J. (1991) *Weighing Goods*. Oxford: Blackwell.

Brueckner, M. and D. Ross (2010) *Under Corporate Skies: a struggle between people, place and profit*. Fremantle: Fremantle Press.

Bundorf, K. and V. R. Fuchs (2008) 'Public support for national health insurance: the roles of attitudes and beliefs', *Forum for Health Economics and Policy*, 10 (1) ('Frontiers in Health Policy Research'): Article 4, http://www.bepress.com/fhep/10/1/4, accessed June 2011.

Cato Institute (nd) 'Individual liberty, free markets and peace', http://www.cato.org/about.php, accessed June 2011.

CBS News (2009) 'Steele calls Obama's health plan socialism', http://www.cbsnews.com/stories/2009/07/20/politics/main5174417.shtml, accessed June 2011.

Chakravarti, A. (2005) *Aid, Institutions and Development*. Cheltenham: Edward Elgar.

Chavez, H. (2009) 'Mision Barrio Adentro', speech, 2 June 2009, http://www.barrioadentro.gov.ve/, accessed June 2011.

Chomsky, A. (2000) '"The threat of a good example": health and revolution in Cuba' in J. Y. Kim, J. V. Millen, A. Irwin and J. Gershman (eds), *Dying for Growth*. Monroe, Maine: Common Courage Press.

Coburn, D. (2000) 'Income inequality, social cohesion and the health status of populations: the role of neoliberalism', *Social Science and Medicine* 51: 135–46.

Cockburn, A. (2005) 'How Coca-Cola gave back to Plachimada', *Counterpunch* (16–17 April), http://www.counterpunch.org/cock burn04162005.html, accessed June 2011.

Cohen, P. (1997) 'Crack in the Netherlands: effective social policy is effective drug policy' in C. Reinarman and H. G. Levine (eds), *Crack in America*. Berkeley CA: University of California Press.

Cooper, R. S., J. F. Kennelly and P. Ordunez-Garcia (2006) 'Health in Cuba', *International Journal of Epidemiology* 35: 817–24.

Coovadia, H., R. Jewkes, P. Barron, D. Saunders and D. McIntyre (2009) 'The health and health system of South Africa: historical roots of current public health challenges', *The Lancet* 374 (9694): 957–9.

Cororaton, C., J. Cockburn and E. Corong (2006) 'Doha scenarios, trade reforms and poverty in the Phillippines: a GCE analysis' in T. W. Hertel and L. A. Winters (eds), *Poverty and the WTO*. Washington DC: World Bank.

Costello, I., M. Abbas *et al.* (2009) 'Managing the health effects of climate change', *The Lancet* 373 (9676): 1693–733.

Council of the European Union (2010) 'Council conclusions on tax and development: cooperating with developing countries in promoting good governance in tax matters', press release, 14 June, http://www.consilium.europa.eu/uedocs/cms_data/docs/pressdata/EN/foraff/115145.pdf, accessed June 2011.

Council of Canadians (2011) 'Kerala, India to fine Coca-Cola for damage to local water', 23 February, http://www.canadians.org/campaignblog/?p=6536, accessed June 2011.

Culyer, A. J. (1988) 'Inequality of health services is, in general, desirable' in D. Green (ed.), *Acceptable Inequalities*. London: IEA Health Unit.

—— (ed.) (1991) *The Economics of Health*. Aldershot: Edward Elgar.

Daily Mail (2010) 'McDonald's, KFC and Pepsi to help write government policy on obesity and diet-related disease', 13 November, http://www.dailymail.co.uk/news/article-1329395/McDonalds-KFC-Pepsi-help-set-government-health-policy-obesity.html#ixzz1Q4UNsfTi, accessed June 2011.

Deaton, A. (2003) 'Health, inequality, and economic development', *Journal of Economic Literature* 41: 113–58.

Democratic Alliance (2009) 'NHI will prove disastrous for South Africa – DA', http://www.politicsweb.co.za/politicsweb/view/politicsweb/en/page71619?oid=132732&sn=Detail, accessed June 2011.

Department of Health (2011) *National Health Insurance in South Africa*. Pretoria: Department of Health.

DHSS (1976) *The RAWP Report*. London: Department of Health and Social

Security, http://www.ncbi.nlm.nih.gov/pubmed?term=%22DixonJ%22%5BAuthor%5D.

Dixon, J. and H. G. Welch (1991) 'Priority setting: lessons from Oregon', *The Lancet* 337 (8746): 891–4.

Drain, P. K. and M. Barry (2010) 'Fifty years of US embargo: Cuba's health outcomes and lessons', *Science* 328 (5978): 572–3.

Dreze, J. and A. Sen (1989) *Hunger and Public Action*. Oxford: Oxford University Press.

—— (2002) *India: development and participation*. Oxford: Oxford University Press.

Dworkin, R. (1989) 'Liberal community', *California Law Review* 77 (3): 479–504.

Elamon, J., R. W. Franke and B. Ekbal (2004) 'Decentralization of health services: the Kerala people's campaign', *International Journal of Health Services* 34 (4): 681–708.

Emini, C., A. Cockburn and B. Decaluwe (2006) 'The poverty impacts of the Doha round in Cameroon: the role of tax policy', in T. W. Hertel and L. A. Winters (eds), *Poverty and the WTO*. Washington DC: World Bank.

Enthoven, A. (1985) *Reflections on the Management of the NHS*. London: Nuffield Trust.

—— (2006) 'Introducing market forces into health care: a tale of two countries', http://web.worldbank.org/WBSITE/EXTERNAL/COUNTRIES/AFRICAEXT/EXTAFRHEANUTPOP/0,,contentMDK:20775956~menuPK:1108504~pagePK:34004173~piPK:34003707~theSitePK:717020~isCURL:Y,00.html, accessed August 2011.

Epstein, H. (2002) 'The hidden cause of AIDS', *New York Review of Books* 49: 8.

Evans, R. G. (1990) 'The dog in the night-time: medical practice variations and health policy' in T. F. Andersen and G. Mooney (eds), *The Challenges of Medical Practice Variations*. Basingstoke: Macmillan.

—— (1997) 'Going for the gold: the redistributive agenda behind market-based health care reform', *Journal of Health Politics, Policy and Law* 22 (2): 427–65.

—— (2008) 'Thomas McKeown, meet Fidel Castro: physicians, population health and the Cuban paradox', *Health Care Policy* 3 (4): 21–32.

Evans, R. G. and G. L. Stoddart (2003) 'Models for population health: consuming research, producing policy?', *American Journal of Public Health* 93 (3): 371–9.

Faith, Family, Freedom Alliance (nd) 'The free market: cornerstone of a free society', http://www.fffa.us/position-papers/the-free-market-cornerstone-of-1/, accessed June 2011.

Foundation of Gaia (nd) 'Transnational corporations', http://www.

foundation-for-gaia.org/index.php?option=com_content&view=articl e&id=59&Itemid=85, accessed June 2011.

Freedman, L. (nd) 'Achieving the MDGs: health systems as core social institutions', http://ipsnews.net/indepth/MDGGoal5/MDG5%20Freed man.pdf, accessed June 2011.

Fuchs, V. R. (1974) *Who Shall Live?* New York NY: Basic Books.

——(1996) 'Economics, values and health care reform', *American Economic Review* 86 (1): 1–24.

—— (2011) *Who Shall Live?* (second edition). London: World Scientific Publications.

Fukuyama, F. (1992) *The End of History and the Last Man.* London: Penguin.

Galbraith, J. (1996) *The Good Society: the humane agenda.* New York NY: Mariner Books.

Gilson, L. (2003) 'Trust and health care as a social institution', *Social Science and Medicine* 6 (67): 1452–68.

Glasner, P. (2001) 'Rights or rituals? Why juries can do more harm than good', *Participatory Learning and Action Notes* 40 (February): 43–5. London: International Institute for Environment and Development.

Global Governance Watch (nd) 'Health and intellectual property: the WTO and TRIPS Agreement', http://www.globalgovernancewatch. org/environment_and_health/health-and-intellectual-property--the-wto-and-trips-agreement, accessed June 2011.

Goklany, I. M. (2011) 'Could biofuel policies increase death and disease in developing countries?', *Journal of American Physicians and Surgeons* 16 (1): 9–13.

Grobler, J. (2009) 'Testing democracy: which way is South Africa going?', http://www.scribd.com/doc/31603161/State-of-Democracy-in-South-Africa, accessed June 2011.

Gupta, S. and E. Cohen (2010) 'Study raises questions about industry funded trials', CNN Health, http://thechart.blogs.cnn.com/2010/08/02/ study-questions-industry-funded-trials/, accessed August 2011.

Gwatkin, D. (2001) 'Poverty and inequalities in health within developing countries: filling the information gap' in D. Leon and G. Walt (eds), *Poverty Inequality and Health.* Oxford: Oxford University Press.

Hamilton, C. (2003) *Growth Fetish.* Sydney: Allen and Unwin.

Hamilton, C. and C. Downie (2007) *University Capture.* Canberra: Australia Institute.

Hansen, J., M. Sato, P. Kharecha, B. Beerling *et al.* (2008) 'Target atmospheric CO_2: where should humanity aim?' *Open Atmosphere Science Journal* 2: 217–31.

Harper, T. A. and G. Mooney (2010) 'Prevention before profits: a levy on food and alcohol advertising', *Medical Journal of Australia* 192 (7)

400–2.

Harvey, D. (2005) *A Brief History of Neoliberalism*. Oxford: Oxford University Press.

Health Poverty Action (2011) 'Key facts: intellectual property and health', http://www.healthpovertyaction.org/policy/trade-and-health/intellectual-property-and-health/key-facts-intellectual-property-and-health/, accessed June 2011.

Hegel, G. W. F. (1820) *The Philosophy of Right*, http://www.marxists.org/archive/marx/works/1843/critique-hpr/intro.htm, accessed August 2011.

Hertel, T. and L. Winters (2006) *Poverty and the WTO*. Washington DC: Palgrave Macmillan and World Bank.

Hirschfeld, K. (2010) 'Cuban health care: consider the source', *Science* 329 (6 August): 627–8.

Hodgson, G. M. (2008) 'An institutional and evolutionary perspective on health economics', *Cambridge Journal of Economics* 32 (2): 235–56.

Hughes, D. (2011) 'Can the government's "responsibility deal" work?', 20 March, http://www.bbc.co.uk/news/health-12776161, accessed June 2011.

Hunter, D. (2011) 'Change of government: one more big bang. Health care reform in England's National Health Service', *International Journal of Health Services* 41 (1): 159–74.

Independent Evaluation Group (2009) *Improving Effectiveness and Outcomes for the Poor*. Washington DC: World Bank.

Irwin, A. and E. Scali (2005) 'Action on the social determinants of health: learning from previous experiences', background paper prepared for the Commission on Social Determinants of Health, http://www.who.int/social_determinants/resources/action_sd.pdf, accessed June 2011.

Jan, S. (2003) 'A perspective on the analysis of credible commitment and myopia in health sector decision making', *Health Policy* 63 (3): 269–78.

Jensen, U. J. (1987) *Practice and Progress: a theory for the modern healthcare system*. London: Blackwell Scientific Publications.

Jolly, R. (1991) 'Adjustment with a human face: a UNICEF record and perspective on the 1980s', *World Development* 19: 1807–21.

Jones-Lee, M. (2002) 'Valuing safety in road project evaluation', *Applied Health Economics and Health Policy* 1 (3): 115–17.

Kashefi, E. and M. Mort (2004) 'Grounded citizens' juries', *Health Expectations* 7: 1–13.

Kasper, W. and M. E. Streit (1998) *Institutional Economics*. Cheltenham: Edward Elgar.

Katz, A. (2007) 'The Sachs Report: investing in health for economic development – or increasing the size of the crumbs from the rich man's table?' in V. Navarro (ed.), *Neoliberalism, Globalization and Inequalities*. New York NY: Baywood.

Kelly, J. and Graziani, R. (2004) 'International trends in company tax rates: implications for Australia's company income tax', *Economic Roundup*, Australian Treasury, Spring, pp 23–47. Available at http://www.treasury.gov.au/documents/930/html/docshell.asp?URL=02_International.asp, accessed June 2011.

Klein, N. (2007) *The Shock Doctrine*. London: Allen Lane.

Kristiansen, I. S. and G. Mooney (2004) *Evidence Based Medicine: in its place*. London: Routledge.

Kuntz, D. (1996) 'Statement from the American Public Health Association', http://www.cubasolidarity.net/apha.html, accessed June 2011.

Labour Party (1945) *1945 Labour Party Election Manifesto. Let Us Face the Future: a Declaration of Labour Policy for the Consideration of the Nation*, http://www.labour-party.org.uk/manifestos/1945/1945-labour-manifesto.shtml, accessed June 2011.

Lansley, A. (2010) 'A healthier nation', Policy Green Paper No 12. London: Conservative Party.

Laski, H. (1933) *Democracy in Crisis*. Chapel Hill: University of North Carolina Press.

Le Grand, J., N. Mays and J. Dixon (1998) 'The reforms; success or failure or neither?' in J. Le Grand, N. Mays and J.-A. Mulligan (eds), *Learning from the NHS Internal Market*. London: King's Fund.

Lenton, T., H. Held, *et al.* (2008) 'Tipping elements in the Earth's climate system', *Proceedings of the National Academy of Sciences of the United States of America* 105 (6): 1786–93.

Lexchin, J., L. Bero, B. Djulbegovic and O. Clark (2003) 'Pharmaceutical industry sponsorship and research outcome and quality: systematic review', *British Medical Journal* 326: 1167–70.

MacAskill, E. (2011) 'Barack Obama acts to ease US embargo on Cuba', *The Guardian*, 15 January, http://www.guardian.co.uk/world/2011/jan/15/barack-obama-us-embargo-cuba, accessed June 2011.

Macintyre, K. C. E. and J. Hadad (2002) 'Cuba' in B. J. Fried and L. M. Gaydos (eds), *World Health Systems: Challenges and Perspectives*. Chicago IL: Health Administration Press.

Mackintosh, M. (2007) 'International migration and extreme health inequality: robust arguments and institutions for international redistribution in health care' in D. McIntyre and G. Mooney (eds), *The Economics of Health Equity*. Cambridge: Cambridge University Press.

Mackintosh, M. and M. Koivusalo (2005) 'Health systems and commercialisation: in search of good sense' in M. Mackintosh and M. Koivusalo (eds), *Commercialisation of Health Care*. Basingstoke: Macmillan and UNRISD.

Macpherson, C. B. (1973) *Democratic Theory*. Oxford: Clarendon Press.

Maggiolini, P. and K. Nanini (nd) 'Ethical meaning of the re-emerging thought about "civil economy" in Italy', http://www.ebenspain.org/docs/Papeles/XV/MaggioliniNanini.pdf, accessed June 2011.

Marmot, M. (2006) 'Health in an unequal world', *The Lancet* 368 (9): 2081–94.

Marshall, T. H. (1950) *Citizenship and Social Class and Other Essays.* Cambridge: Cambridge University Press.

Mason, B. (2003) 'US blocks cheap drugs for undeveloped world', January 2003, http://www.wsws.org/articles/2003/jan2003/drug-j17_prn.shtml, accessed June 2011.

McIntyre, D. (2010) 'Should we pursue a universal health system or something else in South Africa?', SHIELD Policy Brief, no. 2, http://uct-heu.s3.amazonaws.com/wp-content/uploads/2010/10/SHIELD-Policy-Brief-2_Should-we-pursue-a-universal-health-system.pdf, accessed June 2011.

McNulty, C. (2009) 'A look at the Venezuelan healthcare system', http://venezuelanalysis.com/analysis/4566, accessed June 2011.

McMichael, A. J., D. Campbell-Lendrum *et al.* (2004) 'Global climate change' in M. Ezzati, A. D. Lopez, A. Rodgers and C. J. L. Murray (eds), *Comparative Quantification of Health Risks: global and regional burden of disease attributable to selected major risk factors*, Volume 2. Geneva: WHO.

MercoPress (2011) 'WTO says Doha round faces collapse unless agreement is reached before 2012', 27 May, http://en.mercopress.com/2011/05/27/wto-says-doha-round-faces-collapse-unless-agreement-is-reached-before-2012, accessed August 2011.

Minnesota Medical Association (2004) Resolution no. 104, September, http://www.mnmed.org/LinkClick.aspx?fileticket=%2Bd0Nq0qjJCA%3D&tabid=2025, accessed June 2011.

Modus Operandi (2007) 'Water: the Coca-Cola company in Kerala', http://www.openrim.org/IMG/pdf/Case_study_Coca_Cola.pdf, accessed June 2011.

Mooney, G. (2005) 'Addiction and social compassion', *Drug and Alcohol Review* 24 (2): 137–41.

—— (2009) *Challenging Health Economics.* Oxford: Oxford University Press.

—— (2010) 'Citizens' juries', www.gavinmooney.com, accessed June 2011.

Mooney, G. and S. Blackwell (2004) 'Whose health service is it anyway?', *Medical Journal of Australia* 180: 76–8.

Mooney, G. and L. Gilson (2009) 'The economic situation in South Africa and health inequities', *The Lancet* 374 (9693): 858–9.

Mooney, G. and E. Russell (2003) 'Equity in health care: the need for a new paradigm?' in A. Scott, A. Maynard and R. Elliott (eds), *Advances in Health Economics.* Chichester: Wiley.

Mukherjee-Reed, A. (2011) 'Food security as if women mattered: a story from Kerala', http://www.twnside.org.sg/title2/susagri/2011/susagri145.htm, accessed June 2011.

Muller, J. Z. (2003) *The Mind and the Market: capitalism in Western thought.* New York NY: Anchor Books.

Munro, D. (2004) 'Method in political economy: a comment', *Journal of Australian Political Economy* 54: 146–7.

Muntaner, C., R. M. Salazar, J. Benach and F. Armada (2006) 'Venezuela's Barrio Adentro: an alternative to neoliberalism in health care' in V. Navarro (ed.), *Neoliberalism, Globalization, and Inequalities: consequences for health and quality of life.* New York NY: Baywood.

Murray, C. and A. Lopez (1996) *Global Burden of Disease.* Cambridge MA: Harvard University Press.

Narayana, D. (2007) 'High cost achievements and good access to health care at great cost: the emerging Kerala situation' in S. Haddad, E. Baris and D. Narayana (eds), *Safeguarding the Health Sector in Times of Macroeconomic Instability.* Ottawa: IDRC.

Navarro, V. (ed.) (2002) *The Political Economy of Social Inequalities.* New York NY: Baywood.

—— (ed.) (2007a) *Neoliberalism, Globalization and Inequalities.* New York NY: Baywood.

—— (2007b) 'What is a national health policy?', *International Journal of Health Services* 37 (1): 1–14.

—— (2011) 'The importance of politics in policy', *Australian and New Zealand Journal of Public Health* 35 (4): 313.

New York Times (2011) 'Health care reform', http://topics.nytimes.com/top/news/health/diseasesconditionsandhealthtopics/health_insurance_and_managed_care/health_care_reform/index.html, accessed June 2011.

Nussbaum, M. (2001) *Upheavals of Thought.* Cambridge: Cambridge University Press.

Ochoa, F. R. and C. M. Lopez Pardo (1997) 'Economy, politics, and health status in Cuba', *International Journal of Health Services* 27 (4): 791–807.

OECD (2011) 'Growing income inequality in OECD countries: what drives it and how can policy tackle it?', OECD Forum on Tackling Inequality, Paris, 2 May, http://www.oecd.org/dataoecd/32/20/47723414.pdf.

Pamuk, O. (2001) 'The anger of the damned', *New York Review of Books*, http://www.nybooks.com/articles/archives/2001/nov/15/the-anger-of-the-damned/, accessed June 2011.

Pan American Health Organization (PAHO) (2006) *Mission Barrio Adentro: the right to health and social inclusion in Venezuela.* Caracas: PAHO, http://www.paho.org/English/DD/PUB/BA_ENG_TRANS.pdf, accessed June 2011.

Parrott, S. and C. Godfrey (2004) 'Economics of smoking cessation', *British Medical Journal* 328: 947–9.

Pascal, B. (nd) (1623–62) *Thoughts*. Selection in The Harvard Classics, pp. 1909–14, http://www.bartleby.com/48/1/14.html, accessed June 2011.

Pear, R. (2009) 'Doctors' group opposes Public Insurance Plan', *New York Times*, 10 June.

Pécoul, B., P. Chirac, P. Trouiller and J. Pinel (1999) 'Access to essential drugs in poor countries: a lost battle?', *Journal of the American Medical Association* 281 (4): 361–7.

People's Health Movement (2011) 'Bill Gates invitation to World Health Assembly', http://www.phmovement.org/en/node/72, accessed June 2011.

Pogge, T. (2008) 'Health care reform that works for the US and for the world's poor', http://www.ghgj.org/Pogge_Health%20Care%20Reform. pdf, accessed June 2011.

Polanyi, K. (1957 [1944]) *The Great Transformation: the political and economic origins of our time.* Boston: Beacon Press.

Preventative Health Taskforce (2009a) *Australia: The Healthiest Country by 2020 – National Preventative Health Strategy – Overview.* Canberra: Preventative Health Taskforce, http://www.preventativehealth.org.au/ internet/preventativehealth/publishing.nsf/Content/nphs-overview.

—— (2009b) *Australia: The Healthiest Country by 2020 – Technical Report No 1: Obesity in Australia: a need for urgent action.* Canberra: Preventative Health Taskforce, http://www.preventativehealth.org.au/ internet/preventativehealth/publishing.nsf/Content/tech-obesity.

Public Citizen (2011) 'Leaked cables show US tried, failed to organize against Ecuador compulsory licensing', 10 May, http://www.citizen. org/leaked-cables-show-US-tried-failed-to-organize-against-ecuador-compulsory-licensing, accessed June 2011.

Public Records Office (1945) 'Memorandum by the Minister of Health', CAB 129/3. London: Public Records Office.

Rabin, M. (1993) 'Incorporating fairness into game theory and economics', *American Economic Review* 83: 1281–302.

Raffer, K. and H. W. Singer (2001) *The Economic North South Divide: six decades of unequal development.* Cheltenham: Edward Elgar.

Raghavan, C. (2000) 'NGOs campaign against basmati patents', http://www.twnside.org.sg/title/2129.htm, accessed June 2011.

Ramesh, R. (2010) 'Report condemns swine flu experts' ties to big pharma', *The Guardian*, 4 June, http://www.guardian.co.uk/business/2010/ jun/04/swine-flu-experts-big-pharmaceutical, accessed June 2011.

Rand Corporation (2007) 'Conceptualizing and defining public health emergency preparedness', 7 April, http://www.news-medical.net/ ?id=23254, accessed June 2011.

Ranson, K., R. Beaglehole, C. M. Correa, Z. Mirza, K. Buse and N. Drager (2002) 'The public health implications of multilateral trade agreements' in K. Lee, K. Buse and S. Fustukian (eds), *Health Policy in a Globalising World*. Cambridge: Cambridge University Press.

Rawls, J. (1971) *A Theory of Justice*. Oxford: Oxford University Press.

Redman, J. (2008) 'Dirty is the new clean: a critique of the World Bank's Strategic Framework for Development and Climate Change, Sustainable Energy and Economy Network', Institute for Policy Studies, www.ips-dc.org/files/287/dirtyisnewcleanFINAL.pdf, accessed June 2011.

Reich, M. (2000) 'The global drug gap', *Science* 287 (5460):1979–81.

Reinhardt, U. (1992) 'Reflections on the meaning of efficiency: can efficiency be separated from equity?', *Yale Law and Policy Review* 10 (2): 302–15.

Reynolds, T. (2001) 'Industry-funded versus publicly funded trials: are the standards the same?', *Journal of the National Cancer Institute* 93 (21): 1590–2.

Ridley, R. (2001) 'Malaria drug development', report from a symposium held at the 2001 AAAS annual meeting, San Francisco, 17 February, http://www.aaas.org/international/africa/malaria/ridley.html, accessed June 2011.

Ritter, D. (2011) 'Australian of the Year maybe, but business is business', *Crikey*, 1 February, http://www.crikey.com.au/2011/02/01/australian-of-the-year-maybe-but-business-is-business, accessed June 2011.

Robinson, J. (1972) 'Consumers' sovereignty in a planned economy' in A. Nove and D. M. Nuti (eds), *Socialist Economics*. Harmondsworth: Penguin.

Romanow, R. (2002) 'Commission on the Future of Health Care in Canada', The Romanow Commission, http://www.hc-sc.gc.ca/hcs-sss/com/fed/romanow/index-eng.php, accessed June 2011.

Ross, E. (2011) 'How drug companies' PR tactics skew the presentation of medical research', 20 May, http://www.guardian.co.uk/science/2011/may/20/drug-companies-ghost-writing-journalism, accessed June 2011.

Roxon, N. (2009) Speech to the Australian Food and Grocery Council Dinner, 28 October, http://www.health.gov.au/internet/ministers/publishing.nsf/Content/sp-yr09-nr-nrsp281009.htm, accessed June 2011.

Sen, A. (1977) 'Rational fools: a critique of the behavioral foundations of economic theory', *Philosophy and Public Affairs* 6 (4): 317–44.

—— (1992) *Inequality Re-Examined*. Oxford: Clarendon Press.

—— (1999) *Development as Freedom*. Oxford: Oxford University Press.

—— (2001) 'Economic progress and health' in D. Leon and G. Walt (eds), *Poverty, Inequality and Health*. Oxford: Oxford University Press.

Shiell, A. and G. Mooney (2002) 'A framework for determining the extent of public financing of programs and services', Discussion Paper No. 6, Commission on the Future of Health Care in Canada. Ottawa: Government of Canada Publications.

Sierra, J. A. (nd) 'History of Cuba. Economic embargo timeline', http://www.historyofcuba.com/history/funfacts/embargo.htm, accessed June 2011.

Sivaraman, M. (1998) 'Learning from Cuba', *Frontline* 15 (8) (11–24 April), http://www.hindu.com/fline/fl1508/15080570.htm, accessed June 2011.

South African Government (1996) Constitution of the Republic of South Africa, http://www.info.gov.za/documents/constitution/, accessed June 2011.

Spartacus Educational (nd) John Maynard Keynes, http://www.spartacus.schoolnet.co.uk/TUkeynes.htm, accessed June 2011.

Spiegel, J. M. and A. Yassi (2004) 'Lessons from the margins of globalization: appreciating the Cuban health paradox', *Journal of Public Health Policy* 25 (1): 85–110.

Spritzler, J. (2001) 'Did the Jeffrey Sachs AIDS speech deserve applause?', http://www.newdemocracyworld.org/old/aids.htm, accessed June 2011.

Stark, J. (2009) 'How the fast food industry took a leaf out of tobacco's book', *The Age*, 9 August, http://www.theage.com.au/national/how-fast-food-took-a-leaf-out-of-tobaccos-book-20090808-edm7.html, accessed June 2011.

Stiglitz. J. (2003) *Globalization and Its Discontents.* London: Norton.

—— (2006) 'Scrooge and intellectual property rights', *BMJ* 333:1279, http://www.bmj.com/content/333/7582/1279, accessed June 2011

Stolberg, S. and K. Sack (2011) 'Obama backs easing state health law mandates', *The New York Times*, 28 February, http://www.nytimes.com/2011/03/01/us/politics/01health.html?sq=health%20care%20reform&st=cse&scp=6&pagewanted=print, accessed June 2011.

Stuckler, D., S. Basu and M. McKee (2011) 'International Monetary Fund and aid displacement', *International Journal of Health Services* 41 (1): 67–76.

Suchitra, M. (2009) 'Kerala spearheads community-care revolution', *Appropriate Technology* 36 (2): 49–51.

Swilling, M. (2010) 'Intelligent power: SA is throwing it all away', *Cape Times*, 7 April.

Taylor, C. (1991) *The Malaise of Modernity.* Toronto: Anansi.

The Editors (2009) 'What is socialism in 2009?', *The New York Times*, 14 September, http://roomfordebate.blogs.nytimes.com/2009/09/14/what-is-socialism-in-2009/, accessed June 2011.

The India Daily (2011) 'Kerala okays a bill to penalise Coca Cola', 25 February, http://www.theindiadaily.com/kerala-okays-a-bill-to-penalise-coca-cola/, accessed June 2011.

The Lancet (nd) 'The health benefits of tackling climate change: an executive summary for *The Lancet* Series', http://download.thelancet.com/flatcontentassets/series/health-and-climate-change.pdf, accessed June 2011.

The Lancet (2009) 'Editorial: A Commission on climate change', *The Lancet* 373 (9676): 1659, http://download.thelancet.com/pdfs/journals/lancet/PIIS0140673609609223.pdf, accessed 30 January 2012.

The New Age (2011) 'SA urges "democracy" process to name IMF boss', 31 May, http://www.thenewage.co.za/19304-1007-53-SA_urges_'democracy'_process_to_name_IMF_boss, accessed June 2011.

Titmuss, R. (1970) *The Gift Relationship: from human blood to social policy*. London: New Press.

UNDP (1999) *Human Development Report 1999*, Oxford: Oxford University Press, http://hdr.undp.org/en/media/hdr_1999_front.pdf, accessed June 2011.

Vanberg, V. J. (1994) *Rules and Choice in Economics*. London: Routledge.

Via Campesina (2008) 'Collapse of WTO negotiation', press release, 6 August, http://www.viacampesina.org/en/index.php?option=com_content&view=article&id=593:release-of-via-campesina-on-collapse-of-wto-negotiation&catid=21:food-sovereignty-and-trade&Itemid=38, accessed June 2011.

Vick, S. and A. Scott (1998) 'Agency in health care: examining patients' preferences for attributes of the doctor–patient relationship', *Journal of Health Economics* 17: 587–605.

Wagerup Medical Practitioners' Forum (2005), Submission to the Environmental Review and Management Program on the Wagerup Refinery Unit Three Expansion, http://www.abc.net.au/4corners/content/2005/wagerup_med_submission.pdf, accessed June 2011.

Westhoff, W. W., R. Rodriguez, C. Cousin and R. J. McDermott (2010) 'Cuban healthcare providers in Venezuela: a case study', *Public Health* 124 (9): 519–24.

Weston, D. (2011) 'The Political Economy of Global Warming', PhD thesis, Curtin University, Perth.

WHO (2000) *The World Health Report 2000*. Geneva: World Health Organization.

—— (2001) 'Investing in health for economic development'. Report of the Commission on Macroeconomics and Health, chaired by Jeffrey D. Sachs. Geneva: WHO.

—— (2008) 'Closing the gap in a generation: health equity through action on the social determinants of health'. Report of the Commission on Social Determinants of Health, http://www.who.int/social_determinants/thecommission/finalreport/en/, accessed June 2011.

Wilkinson, R. (2005) *The Impact of Inequality*. London: Routledge.

Wilkinson, R. and K. Pickett (2006) 'Income inequality and population health: a review and explanation of the evidence', *Social Science and Medicine* 62: 1768–84.

—— (2010) *The Spirit Level*. London: Allen Lane.

Williams, A. (1993) 'Priorities and research strategy in health economics for the 1990s', *Health Economics* 2 (4): 295–302.

Williamson, J. (2002) 'What Washington means by policy reform' in J. Williamson (ed.) *Latin American Adjustment: how much has happened* (original edition 1990, updated November 2002). Washington DC: Peterson Institute for International Economics.

World Bank (1993) *Investing in Health*. Washington DC: World Bank.

—— (2011) 'Health expenditure', http://data.worldbank.org/indicator/SH.XPD.TOTL.ZS, accessed August 2011.

WTO (2001) Ministerial Declaration, Doha WTO Ministerial 2001, WT/MIN(01)/DEC/1, 20 November, http://www.wto.org/English/thewto_e/minist_e/min01_e/mindecl_e.htm, accessed June 2011.

Zamagni, S. (2010) 'Non-profit organizations, democratic stakeholding and civil development', presentation to WINGS forum 2010, 18–20 November, Como, Italy, http://www.wingsweb.org/download/2010%20Forum/Plenary_Italian_Philanthropy_Zamagni.pdf, accessed June 2011.

Zarri, L. (2006) 'Happiness, morality and game theory', Working Paper Series 37, Department of Economics, University of Verona.

Index

Printed and bound by CPI Group (UK) Ltd, Croydon, CR0 4YY

11/10/2024

01043584-0001